# THE LOW BACK PAIN-FREE PROGRAM

A STEP-BY-STEP GUIDE TO HELP YOU ACHIEVE A
LIFETIME FREE OF LOWER BACK PAIN!

BY DR. LEO CHOU, DC

# CONTENTS

# A GIFT FOR YOU

## 3 Daily Miracle Exercises: Have Total Control on Lower Back Health

Jumpstart your low back pain recovery journey now!

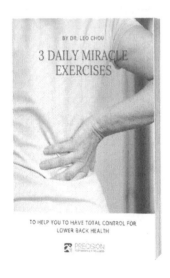

In this 3 Daily Miracle Exercises Guide, you'll learn:

- A shortcut exercise routine to help with low back pain in under 6 minutes.
- The most important key concept is to have a healthy low back.

- The top 3 habits you need to keep the pain away from the low back.

To receive your exercise scan the QR code below or visit - www.precisionperformancecalgary.com/gift

# INTRODUCTION

Imagine it's been a long day at the all-day conference you had to attend as part of your work commitments. It ran late into the evening, and after travelling to the city first thing, you can't wait to hit the hay. There's nothing more satisfying after a hard day, than sinking into the crisp, fresh, super-soft bed that awaits you in your hotel room, *right?*

That is, unless you suffer from low back pain...

For back pain sufferers, we know that allowing the mattress to swallow us up for the night means we'll pay a heavy price the next day, and I'm not just talking about the cost of the hotel room. Even the most luxurious hotels can have a bed that just isn't suitable for anyone who has back issues.

Following their stay, back pain sufferers will face crippling pain the next morning. They may have to roll or chuck themselves out of the bed as the agony can be debilitating. Many suffer stiffness in their lower back, which is often accompanied with a pulling sensation that can travel down the hips and thighs, sometimes reaching right down to the knee. Most sufferers find themselves turning to pain relief medication. While some may try to stretch this, they can still end up waddling around, feeling fragile and struggling to sit or stand, until the pain subsides, whenever that may be.

For some, it's a few hours, but for more severe cases, it could be weeks or several months. Low back pain is a common complaint by many people all over the world and after witnessing its life-limiting effects, I acknowledge that it is time for change. No longer do you have to suffer from low back stiffness – that excruciating shooting pain that runs along the bottom of your spine – or any of the other symptoms that make your physical life difficult.

*It doesn't have to be like that and I call on you to take immediate action!*

Jim Rohn says, *"Take care of your body. It's the only place you have to live,"* (Bhatt, A. 2020) and he has a point there. We have to maintain and sustain our body for life, and we only get one opportunity to do that. So, if you're no longer willing to put up with lower back pain and the suffering it brings, and you are ready for your back to be pain free, you should continue to take action by reading this book.

As a successful chiropractor, and Clinical Director of Precision, Performance and Wellness with a clinic that specializes in holistic sports injuries, I have treated many patients with simple to complex low back pain conditions and have helped them regain functionality. I understand the severity of lower back pain, and believe that with consistency and motivation, people can manage or even heal their low back conditions with minimal effort. That's why I believe it's important to allow my patients to have access to resources for self-care when dealing with lower back pain injuries at home.

Low back pain is much more common than you may think, and sufferers often just put up with the physical pain rather than remedying it. People constantly make excuses to justify it, for instance, we acknowledge that we shouldn't have sat in an uncomfortable chair all day at the office, or maybe we went a little crazy at the gym. We often use these excuses to explain the condition and then we don't take action to prevent or correct the issues.

It may surprise you to hear that over 31 million Americans suffer with low back pain at any one time, and yet, many problems are self-manageable. The purpose of this book is to encourage sufferers to take action against their low back pain in a way that can remedy the issue. Through the use of self-care methods, exercise routines, and holistic healthcare strategies, you can learn to manage your condition, which results in your back becoming pain free.

In order to remedy any back issues, we need to get to the root of the problem, and to do this, we must first explore what low back pain is exactly. Then, we must find out what caused the pain or injury in the first place. This is something we'll explore in detail throughout this book. Most low back pain issues can be self-managed in a simple yet inexpensive way that does not consume too much of your time or energy. In the long-term, this could prevent more serious issues.

I personally believe that most low back pain issues can be easily resolved if we respond quickly, and more serious issues can be prevented from arising as a result. By increasing awareness and education, many minor back pain issues can be prevented from spiraling out of control. So many of my clients have commented, *"If I only knew this sooner..."*.

We all know that certain issues and conditions are avoidable and can be remedied, especially in the earlier stages. I'm willing to share my knowledge and expertise, and all those things I wish I knew when I first suffered with severe low back pain. As a healthcare professional, I recognize the value that such education and awareness offers. After all, I embarked on a career in healthcare because I'm passionate about improving and enriching the lives of others.

Back pain can be frustrating as well as agonizing but early knowledge of issues that can occur puts the power and ownership back into your hands. We are all independent and self-sufficient, and while education and awareness is power, the ability to take control of your health and physical fitness lies within you.

As I work side-by-side with other healthcare professionals in a multidisciplinary clinic, I am able to share the wealth of knowledge shared with me on a daily basis by physiotherapists, massage therapists, psychologists, naturopaths, family doctors, and acupuncturists, which has only enriched and strengthened my personal and professional experience when it comes to low back issues.

If you're tired of the pain, frustrated by the stiffness, and are ready to target your low back pain issues, then you must head over to chapter 1, so we can focus on what low back pain is and its causes.

*Are you ready to take action against your low back pain?*

If yes, then you MUST read on. Make no mistake, what I'm about to share with you has the potential to change your life. It's down to you to make that happen!

*Let's do this!*

# WHAT YOU NEED TO KNOW ABOUT LOW BACK PAIN

In order to really understand low back pain, there are some things you need to know. In this chapter, we'll look at the anatomy and consider the different structures in the body, such as the spine, the pelvis, joints and discs, muscles and tendons, ligaments, and nerves. We will then consider how each structure functions and the potential pain and discomfort caused by each if they dysfunction. Sometimes, we suffer from lower back pain and we don't really know why or what to do.

*"Dear back pain please go. I can't stand, neither sit nor bow!!"*

— MRINMOY (BHATT, 2020)

As the quote above suggests, you can't sit, bow, or stand, as each of those things cause us pain. If we don't act, we run the risk of it becoming worse.

The lower back region is at the back of the body and begins just below the ribcage. It is often referred to as the lumbar region. Many people suffer with back pain but it usually passes within a few weeks without them requiring any treatment. This is often a warning sign that you need to take more care of your body, including your lower back. But in order to understand the pains and warning signs, we need to understand our lower back anatomy and become aware of the things that may cause us pain and discomfort. Then, we can aim to prevent them from occurring.

By the end of this chapter, you will understand the anatomical structures involving low back pain and low back pain risk factors. Let's start by reviewing the different parts of the body that form the lower back.

## The Vertebrae and Lumbar Spine

There are 24 vertebrae that run down the center of your back and together make up the spinal column. There are 7 in the neck that make up the cervical spine, 12 in the middle back that make up the thoracic spine, and 5 in the lower back that make up the lumbar spine.

## The Sacroiliac Joint and Pelvis

The sacroiliac joint is often involved with low back pain and dysfunction. The joint connects the base of the spine with the pelvis. The pelvis itself is made up of three bones: the ilium, the ischium, and the pubis.

## The Intervertebral Discs

The intervertebral discs are sometimes referred to as the spinal discs. They provide shock absorbing qualities as they are soft tissue material situated between the vertebrae. The intervertebral discs are made up of two components. The outer layer is tough and is made up of annulus fibrosus. The gelatinous, water-like substance that forms the inner part is the nucleus pulposus. The discs help us to move and bend, and as we rotate, the compression forces them to change shape and act as cushions between the vertebrae. The intervertebral discs also form part of the intervertebral foramen. This is the space, bounded by disc and vertebrae, where the spinal nerves travel.

## Muscles and Tendons

There are muscles and tendons located around the spine that help to stabilize the spinal joints. The tendons connect the muscles to bones and both assist with movements in the back.

The muscles contain individual muscle fibers and are striated in their appearance. Each muscle fiber contracts to produce body movement. In turn, this produces natural waste products which are muscular metabolism products composed of biological acids. Each acid is recycled in the body and rich in blood supply, but if they are not recycled effectively, they can contribute to back pain.

The tendons are different from the muscles because they are made up of collagen and elastin. Collagen and elastin are proteins but unlike muscles, they don't contract. They have much smaller blood supply and do not produce as much waste as the muscles do. The tendons are strong, fibrous connectives that help stabilize during times of movement.

## Ligament and Nerves

The ligaments are similar to tendons, and they too connect and stabilize joints. They are connective tissues which connect the bone to the next bone.

The nerves in the back travel from the central nervous system. Originally, they start in the brain and continue through the spinal cord, which is protected by the spinal column. The spinal cord branches off into nerve roots that exit the spine and transform into spinal nerves. They help the brain to communicate with all structures within the body. There are two types of nerves in the back that we need to focus on: motor nerves and sensory nerves. The motor nerves send signals from the brain to target muscles and tell them when to contract. The sensory nerves are embedded in the vertebrae, joints, ligaments, skin, and muscles. The nerves are located all over the body. They react and then send signals back to the brain so that we can interpret them. For instance, rubbing the back of your hand can produce warmth and feelings of comfort and relaxation.

## Joint Complex

All of the above work together as a complex system. They are a highly dynamic, biological structure. Understanding the anatomy and how each part works is important if you want to begin to prevent or remedy low back pain.

Now that we've explored the different parts of the back that make up the joint complex, you can begin to understand the complexity of back problems. Many back problems can be prevented if we are simply more aware of what causes the issues in the first place. By knowing the warning signs, we can take measures to reduce the likelihood of back pain becoming a long-term issue. *But what causes low back pain?*

In order to move forward and create a deeper understanding of why low back pain occurs and what can cause it, we need to review the risks of low back pain developing.

## Risk Factors for Developing Low Back Pain

There are many reasons why low back pain develops. If you can start to pinpoint the causes or risks, you can treat this early or even prevent it from occurring initially. While low back pain can occur from an activity we complete, sometimes there are more complex issues. By understanding the risks, or how our low back pain is triggered, we can reduce the likelihood of back pain and promote good back care.

## Psychological Factors

There are many psychological factors that can lead to low back pain. Research indicates that anxiety and depression are closely linked to low back pain. This is because of the tension we feel which causes joints to stiffen. Also, when a person is depressed, ahxious, or stressed, they tend to pay less attention to themselves.

They ignore pain and don't focus on the severity therefore allowing the pain to worsen. Sufferers can also have difficulty coping with the pain with many needing medical attention.

## Occupational Risk Factors

Occupational risks include those who have to work on computers regularly and have increased screen-time and those who are performing the same manual tasks or activities repeatedly. Simple tasks such as bending forward can cause issues if performed incorrectly, especially if there is twisting involved too.

Think about your mailman delivering mail, a factory worker who collects the finished product and puts it into a vehicle for shipping, or a mother picking her small child up off the floor. The combination of bending and twisting puts stress on the discs in your back, and eventually, this will lead to a tear. This type of movement can also cause stress to other structural tissues including vertebral ligaments, cartilage, and muscles.

Office workers tend to sit for long periods of time, often with poor posture. They round their back and sometimes tense their shoulders which can result in them becoming stiff. The rounding back posture is often described as creeping in the spine. Sitting is often viewed as being less intense than those who have a more laborious role, which is physically demanding, and yet, it has a similar effect as repetitive manual labor.

## Obesity

The more weight you carry, the more stress your body faces. The physical demands on your back become a strain and increase your chances of injuries. Weight causes both biochemical stress as well as mechanical stress, which affects how your body works as it moves. Two types of fat cells appear in the body. The first type is large and releases pro-inflammatory chemicals into the body. They stimulate our nerve cells for painful sensations. The other type of fat cells is small and are made up from anti-inflammatory immune cells.

## Pregnancy

During pregnancy the body reacts differently and begins to release special hormones into the body. The hormone causes ligaments around the sacroiliac joint to be loose and flexible. This hormone is called Relaxin and its purpose is to help the body adapt in line with the baby's growth but there are some side effects. First of all, it can cause pain in the spine or pelvis. It can also cause instability. While most back pain during pregnancy happens between the fifth and eighth month, for some women it begins as early as eight to twelve weeks.

Weight gain is expected during a healthy pregnancy and women can expect to gain between 25-33 lbs. As with all weight gain, this puts stress on the body and in particular, the spine, which is used to support the weight. In turn, this increases the pressure on joints and nerves in the back and can cause us pain. For a woman, their center shifts during later pregnancy, and this causes changes in posture too. As discussed earlier, poor posture can result in back pain too.

**Smoking**

It may seem crazy that smoking is linked to back pain but there are some key, scientifically-researched reasons that indicate there is a clear link between smoking and low back pain. The correlation between smoking and low back pain is clear and it is important to recognize the relationship.

Smoking creates hormone alterations in the body and such hormonal changes are linked to low back pain. People who smoke and have a chronic cough as a result may also suffer from low back pain. That is because coughing is a mechanical stress to the body, which can result in low back pain. Smoking also has a close link to anxiety and depression. Anxiety and depression are also linked to low back pain as discussed earlier in the chapter.

## Age

The older we get, the more wear and tear our body faces. Experts say that low back pain typically occurs around the ages of 30-50, and with age, muscle elasticity and tone decreases. In addition, our intervertebral discs lose their flexibility and fluid, so there is less cushioning in the spine. Bone density also decreases with age and so does bone strength leading to further concerns of osteoporosis, which can result in fractures. Our ligaments thicken, and this means that the spinal canal becomes narrow which can also compress the nerves in the spine.

## Genetics

There are certain conditions that we can be prone to due to our genetics. An example of a genetic condition that affects the spine includes ankylosing spondylitis. This is a form of arthritis which results in fusion of spinal joints and can reduce mobility in the spine. This is due to the HLA-B gene, which provides instructions for making a type of protein that is an important component in our immune system. Not only does this lead to mobility issues in the spine but it can also cause rigidity.

Throughout this chapter, we have explored the different parts of the body that make up our lower back, which has helped us to begin navigating and understanding our anatomy. While we've looked at some of the physical impacts of back pain, there is so much more to consider. It is important to remember that back pain is often a complex issue and also has effects on both the mind and body due to the impact the pain itself can have on us.

**ACTIVITY - Check in with Yourself**

Think about the warning signs or pain you suffer with when it comes to your lower back and ask yourself the questions listed below:

- What causes discomfort or pain to your back (bending, twisting, etc.)?
- What activities make it worse?
- How does it affect you?
- What risks do you take every day that can make your back pain worse (for example, your job or career, sports, pregnancy, smoking, etc.)?
- On a scale of 1-10 with 10 being the most intense pain and 1 being the lowest, how much pain are you in with your back when it's at its worst?
- What would your life be like if you could

improve, manage, and maintain your lower
back pain?

In the next chapter, we will introduce pain and link it
to the impact it has on the mind and body. By building
a deeper understanding of the different levels of pain as
well as reviewing how pain is produced and perceived,
you will gain broader knowledge of the connection
between both the mind and the body, and how pain
may affect you.

2

---

# UNDERSTANDING PAIN – THE MIND-BODY CONNECTION FOR BEGINNERS

W hen we suffer with pain, we know it's there as it causes us stress and discomfort, but we don't always question how or why the pain occurs. Pain can impact us in many different ways. For example, toothache can alter our mood and affect our eating habits. General pain, like a headache, can make us feel tired and lack energy. Pain can also affect our mind because there is only so much of it we can take before we need help.

When you have low back pain, it can be debilitating as you can struggle to stay mobile, but there are also different intensities of pain to consider as your ability to identify and cope with the pain is an important part of the recovery process. The pain level indicates whether your back issues are long or short term. That's why it's important to understand how the pain is produced and perceived by our body.

Many people report a niggling pain in the base of their spine, running across the pelvis, before they suffer something substantially more painful occurring with their back. These niggling pains are your first warning signs and must not be ignored!

In this chapter, we will explore the concept of pain in our lower back in order to understand it better. We will also focus on identifying the key differences between acute and chronic pain, so we can learn how pain is actually produced in the first place. We will then investigate how the body perceives pain, how it can affect both the mind and body, and how they are both connected.

**Acute Pain to Chronic Pain**

It is time to focus on pain and compare acute pain with chronic pain. Gaining a stronger understanding of the differences in pain can help us effectively and easily manage and maintain any problems or issues in relation to our lower back.

**What is Acute Pain?**

Acute pain is short-term back pain. By short-term, we mean that it may last from a few days to a few weeks but it's likely that it won't continue beyond that so a full, swift recovery can be made. When it comes to pain in your lower back, most clinic referrals are in relation to an acute pain attack but this is often resolved on its own within a few days. The best way to treat an acute pain attack is by resting and by partaking in some self-care. Generally, there is no long-term effect on body function. However, there are occasional cases in which it takes a few months for symptoms to completely disappear. Some people believe they are cured after only a few days but then they go back to their normal activities too soon, which results in a relapse.

## What is Sub-acute Pain?

If your acute pain lasts for longer than a six-week period, it becomes sub-acute. This means that the intensity of the pain may change from a sharp or burning pain to a dull ache (or vice versa), but it's still there and it's still persistent. Therefore, it impacts your day-to-day activities. If the problem is dealt with effectively, it will not have a long-lasting impact.

## What is Chronic Pain?

Chronic pain usually persists on a long-term basis. This means that the pain lasts for longer than 12 weeks and there are often periods of more intense pain too. Around 20% of people who previously suffered from, and have been treated for, acute back pain report that they have developed chronic low back pain with symptoms lasting for around 12 months.

Although pain causes us stress and discomfort, it does not necessarily mean that there is something seriously wrong medically, nor does it mean there is a serious underlying cause. It is possible that issues can be identified and treated easily. In many cases, chronic back pain can be remedied successfully through medical treatment and patients will feel some relief. For others, it means that the pain continues to be persistent, regardless of medical or surgical treatments. Chronic pain that does not subside can affect patients in many different ways as the pain is persistent and intense.

Chronic pain is often described as being multidimensional and that's because of the different effects it has on its sufferers. Chronic pain sufferers often experience psychological, biological, and physiological processes which link together to form your final response to the pain you're feeling. The psychological distress brought on by pain can be much worse for people who already suffer with anxiety and depression as they often perceive pain in a more severe way. Anyone who suffers from anxiety and depression are classed as high-risk when it comes to low back pain because the level of pain perceived does not necessarily conform with the physical damage to tissue. Often, the pain continues to persist even after the physical damage has improved.

## The Cycle of Chronic Pain

People who suffer from chronic pain tend to fall into the chronic pain cycle but it's important that we don't get stuck in this over and over again as this only escalates the problem. Let's take a look at each part of the cycle as having good knowledge of this allows you to break free and seek the correct treatment from the beginning:

1. **Elevated Focus on Physical Pain** – Our brain becomes focused on the physical pain we are enduring and we start to believe that the tissue damage is causing us harm, which makes us anxious.

2. **Obsession with the Pain** – As the pain isn't subsiding, the anxiety builds, and we become obsessed with the pain. This leads to social isolation as we begin to limit the things we do, which brings on depression too.

3. **Increased Feelings of Anxiety, Depression, and Fatigue** – Depression and anxiety drain us mentally and we begin to tire much more easily. Such feelings only exacerbate chronic pain. Changes occur within the nervous system and we feel more pain and tend to move less, which only makes things worse.

**4. Physical Impairment Causing Us to Function Inadequately** – The more pain relief we take and the more emotional distress we feel results in further mental and physical impairments. Relationships can suffer as a result, especially if we continuously move in this cycle.

This cycle is easy to fall into but hard to break out of. That's why raising awareness about low back pain and being able to differentiate between both acute and chronic pain is so important. Simply recognizing the steps in the cycle so that we don't follow the never-ending pattern is a great way to handle low back pain in the most effective way.

Finding the right treatment is not always simple. There are different factors in finding the most effective treatment, for instance, it starts with identifying the type of pain you have. In order to identify the type of pain we're suffering from, we need to understand our anatomy. We've covered the anatomy in chapter 1, so you're already on the right track. Pain in the lower back can come from:

- Muscles
- Ligaments
- Tendons
- Discs

- Nerves
- Blood Vessels

If we can identify the root cause of our low back pain, we can begin to look for suitable and effective treatments to ease back pain. We'll focus on relevant treatments later in this book.

## Links Between the Body and the Mind

The mind and body are closely connected. The connection is stronger than most people anticipate but to put it simply, if we don't care for our mental health, our physical health can be affected, and vice-versa.

The relationship between mental and physical has always been intimate. The oldest documentation of this was in the form of images, dating back to 5000-3500 BCE, discussed in the oldest translated text from India, *Hindu Traditions of Vendatism.* Vendatism is regularly linked to meditation. It is a philosophy that originated in India and focuses on spiritual enlightenment but it is one of the earliest known paths to meditation.

Meditation is a modality regularly used in the Science of Life. The Science of Life is sometimes known as Ayurveda, which is a comprehensive and natural health system developed in India during Vedic times. Meditation allows the connection to our inner self. According to Vedic Science, we can activate our physical body by linking it to our inner working consciousness. A lot of research has been done to study meditation and its effect on pain. The purpose of meditation is to connect to one's deeper, inner self and benefit from its mind-healing properties. The research suggests that meditation has a positive impact on both physical and psychological pain, and it also decreases anxiety and depression.

There are many instances when we have to take part in tasks that we are not wholly comfortable with. We may begin with a psychological effect that creates a physiological response. For example, we can tense our body during a stressful event which makes us feel afraid or nervous. Maybe you're getting married and feel nervous about the ceremony in front of family and friends, or maybe you're giving a speech or big presentation at work that you feel nervous or fearful about. You could have a physiological response, such as:

- Sweaty palms
- Loss of appetite
- Goosebumps or hairs standing up on our arms or behind the neck
- A nervous stomach that grumbles or feels tense
- Increased heart rate

Each of these responses indicate that the brain and body are in communication with one another. This is often referred to as the *fight-or-flight* response. You may have heard this phrase before. This is a key part in human evolution. When our ancestors were hunting for food whilst watching out for predators, they taught our bodies to automatically fight to survive. They hunted for food and they escaped predators to stay safe. If they were attacked, their muscles were pumped with blood and they would decide whether to run or fight back. Today, we don't really worry about being preyed upon by large animals but there are occasions when we may find ourselves using those instincts to survive a situation. This includes the times we experience emotional stress which is triggered from having to give a speech or presentation or having to take part in a ceremony in front of others. Emotional stress can be triggered by family issues, financial issues and debt, traffic, work performance, a last-minute project, and many other things which can cause us worry, concern, or irritation. This is when our *fight-or-flight* instincts kick in.

If you already suffer with ongoing mechanical issues with muscles, discs, tendons, or muscles, the tension you feel due to your *fight-or-flight* instincts may aggravate these issues and your symptoms may get worse. If you keep responding, using these instincts over a long period of time, it can cause fatigue and your muscles can weaken as a result. This compromises your musculoskeletal system and its equilibrium. Such emotional stress can also cause generalization of inflammation to body systems, which can cause further pain.

## How Does Pain Get Perceived in the Brain?

We all feel pain differently because we perceive it differently. Pain is an individual feeling rather than a collective one because the experience is different for everyone. Whenever we injure our bodies, we feel pain. This could be from a bruise, a fracture, a tear, a cut, or excessive heat or cold. The cells within the damaged tissues release chemicals into whichever part of the body is facing the body. This could be muscles, tendons, ligaments, and even the bone or skin. Our body then carries these chemicals around, so that they can communicate with other substances within the body that stimulate specialized nerve cells called the nociceptors.

The function of the nociceptors is to detect anything alien within the body that poses a threat or damage to the body. There are many nociceptors that deal with a specific environment, for example, there are some that deal with the heat, cold, and mechanical load to the body. The nociceptors send signals up our spinal cord, through afferent nerve fibers, which carry information to the brain. The brain then responds appropriately to the tissues that are under threat by using its efferent nerve fibers. The process of how we respond to pain can be listed in three steps which differs in individuals:

1. **Our Emotional and Psychophysiological Reactions to Pain** – This is how we deal with pain psychologically and physiologically as we all respond differently.

2. **The Attention We Pay to the Pain Itself** – Some people are able to block-out or ignore pain, while others are not good with pain and suffer aloud. They do as little as possible and can't physically do anything as the pain consumes them. There are lots of responses in between the two extremes.

3. **The Way We View Pain Itself** – While many people learn to live with pain and accept it, others complain about the pain every day and struggle to come to terms with the fact that some pain can be long-term.

Perceiving and dealing with pain is complex because we can all only respond to our own experiences. This sometimes makes it difficult to remedy and treat. Sometimes, it takes trial and error to come up with the most effective treatment. This takes patience and perseverance.

## Gate Control Theory of Pain

As we've already discussed, the mind and body communicate with each other regularly. The Gate Control Theory is often used to explain why massage and touch can help in pain management but there is not enough substantiated research or evidence to suggest the actual 'gate control' exists within the body. However, the idea itself can help you to understand how and why some pain signals travel to the brain while others do not. The gate is a great metaphor that can be used to help others understand why pain fluctuates so much, so it's worth a mention.

The Gate Control Theory focuses on what happens before those pain signals that are travelling up the spinal cord reach your brain. Not all pain signals actually reach the brain because again, this is down to how we perceive pain. The pain messages arrive at the 'nerve gates' which are ultimately the control mechanism that decides whether or not the signals should reach the brain. If the pain is more intense, the signals are passed along quickly, but in other instances, signals may not reach the brain at all.

The nerve gates are situated in the dorsal horn of the spinal cord. Both pain fibers and normal fibers carry information to two different areas within the dorsal horn. Pain fibers are small while normal fibers are large. The pain signals are then transmitted straight to the brain if they are deemed viable and allowed to pass, but if not, the pain gates close and the inhibitory interneurons halt the signals or at least impede them. If the pain gates are closed, it is often because the pain is brief and has now gone.

This concept explains in a simpler way how our body and mind work together to interpret pain and how we should deal with it. Now, it's time to look at different sources of pain so we can really get to the root of the problem.

## Different Sources of Pain

### Physical Pain

Physical pain is when we experience pain in a specific area of the body that we've hurt or injured. The pain is the discomfort we feel. Physical pain is caused by many different things, for example, you could pull a muscle, fracture a bone, or cut your leg or arm.

### Referred Pain

Referred pain is when we experience pain in a particular location but the origin of the pain exists somewhere else. The pain occurs in the wrong place because our body consists of interconnecting sensory nerves that consist of an array of different tissues. For example, a person who has a heart attack may experience pain in the arms or jaw.

## Radiating Pain

Radiating pain is a travelling pain. It occurs in one part of the body but ends in another, spreading over a larger area. For example, if you experience nerve pain that runs from the base of your back over your hip and thigh and down to your knee, the pain could be more prominent and persistent in the knee, but the pain originates in the lower back, from your herniated disc.

## When is Back Pain Serious?

When you have back pain, it can become serious quickly but there are some things you can look out for to ensure you do not ignore the warning signs:

1. When the dull aching pain becomes a sharp, persistent pain.
2. When you suffer with radiating pain.
3. If you begin to suffer from bladder or bowel incontinence.
4. Altered sensations or numbness in the groin area.
5. If you begin to feel weakness or limitations to mobility in your legs.

If you suffer from any of the 5 symptoms above, you should seek advice and guidance from a qualified health professional, especially if the symptoms are persistent.

## ACTIVITY – Beginner's Meditation

While many people love meditation and are already doing this as part of their daily routine, other people shy away from this without even giving it a try. Meditation isn't a quick fix, it's something that takes practice and time. Challenge yourself and try out 10 minutes of meditation for at least the next 7 days (although to feel the full benefits of meditation, you should give yourself much more time).

1. Think of three affirmations that suggest you are where you want to be. For instance, if you find yourself stressing about your back pain, then you could say "I'm happy, healthy, and pain-free."
2. Lay down on your back and get comfortable. Try not to cross your arms or legs.
3. Take three deep breaths and then allow yourself to fall back into your natural breathing pattern.
4. Concentrate on your breathing. Focus on the breath.
5. Let go of anything and everything that's on

your mind and think only of your breathing as you sink deeper into your meditation.

6. Repeat your three affirmations, three times to end your meditation. Use the same affirmations for the 7 days, but after that, if you choose to continue with your meditation, you can change them to serve another purpose.

If you struggle to meditate, try listening to some meditation music or binaural tones. The internet is a great resource! You could also try out some guided meditations to help you stay focused. Meditation certainly takes time and focus but it can help you to clear your mind, check in with yourself, and relieve stress. It relaxes your physical body and your whole nervous system.

In this section, we explored acute and chronic pain and considered the way pain is produced and perceived within our body. Now that you have a stronger understanding of pain, you can begin to look more in depth at chronic pain and how it affects both the person and the healthcare system. Pain has more of an impact than most people realize.

# 3

# CHRONIC PAIN AND HOW TO COPE

S uffering from chronic pain is not a pleasant experience. As mentioned in chapter 2, it does not only affect you physically but also mentally. The issues surrounding chronic pain run so much deeper because chronic pain does not only impact the person who suffers from the pain. It also affects health systems across the world as they attempt to help and guide others into managing their pain and ensure they can access the most appropriate treatment.

In this chapter, we will go more in depth about chronic pain. We will explore how chronic pain affects a person and the different ways to manage it. We will also explore the burden faced by the world health system when it comes to chronic pain.

## Chronic Pain and the Health Care Burden

According to Tracy P. Jackson, Victoria Sutton Stabile, and Kelly McQueen (2014), chronic pain is estimated to affect 10% of the world's population, which is around 60 million people. With this in mind, you can imagine the impact this has on healthcare systems all over the world. In some low and middle-income countries or regions, this figure is closer to 20-25%. There is a close correlation between the pain burden to a healthcare system and the level of income of the area in question. For instance, for low-income countries, the higher the burden of persistent pain, the less likely sufferers are to receive effective treatment, even though pain management is a basic human right under international law and has been since 2004.

The reason that chronic pain is such a burden on healthcare is because of the cause and effect it has on other medical and health issues. For example, if someone suffers with low back pain, it could lead to depression and anxiety as well as mobility issues. Disabling pain can also affect mood, so the patient must be provided with help and guidance in order to manage this effectively. This means a patient is not only dealing with persistent pain but they may also need some different medical treatments. For instance, they may need pain relief medication to relieve their symptoms, different therapies from a chiropractor, physiotherapist, or sports therapist (depending on the cause of the injury), and if they are depressed or anxious, they could require counselling or further medication to help overcome the long-term issue. Medication for depression or anxiety have their own side effects, for instance, sleeping and eating could also be affected which could have further impact on the patient's life, including their work. If income is reduced, as the person is no longer able to work in the same roles or needs time off work to recover, then this can have a financial impact on the patient too.

Jackson, Stabile and McQueen (2014) also reveal that "at least 1-4 percent of the global population also suffers from a 'chronic pain syndrome'... comprising multiple somatic pain complaints and psychological 'distress'." A chronic pain syndrome are things like chronic fatigue, fibromyalgia, somatoform disorder, and neurasthenia, which can all cause widespread pain.

The cost of health in relation to low back pain is huge. In 2021, based on statistics from the U.S., over $300 billion per year on average was spent in relation to low back pain only, and there was an increased demand for benzodiazepines to treat pain and related symptoms like insomnia, anxiety, and pain itself. In addition, there are other costs to consider. Time out of work, long-term disabilities that are formed as a result of chronic pain, mental health interventions and social support, as well as complementary therapies and surgical procedures may need to be considered on top of the initial sum.

Not all countries are able to offer the same care nor do they have the same financial support available. Many people start out with acute pain but due to lack of access or finances ignore their acute pain issues, and this results in persistent and chronic pain becoming a long-term issue or developing into a chronic pain syndrome.

Now that we've explored the global burden of chronic pain, it is time to explore how chronic pain affects a person.

**How Chronic Pain Affects a Person**

Chronic pain affects a person biologically, psychologically, socially, and it also impacts their quality of life and health. Each of these interlink, so for example, a biological effect could have a psychological effect and a psychological effect could have a social impact, and vice-versa. They all impact the quality of life and health aspect of your life too.

Let's look at some examples of the affects chronic pain can have on a person:

- **Biological** – The biological impact of pain includes trauma, nerve damage, illness, injury, infection, and cancer.
- **Psychological** – The psychological impact of pain includes lack of sleep, coping skills, fear, depression, and anxiety.
- **Social** – The social impact of pain includes failing relationships within family, social networks, and at work.
- **Quality of Life and Health** – Pain can also impact social and family function, the physical functioning of your body, life activities, and mental health.

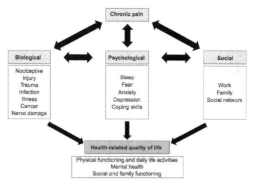

**Figure 1** Biopsychosocial model of pain and consequences on the quality of life.

Research by Maria Duenas, Begona Ojeda, Alejandro Salazar, Juan Antonio Mico, and Inmaculada Failde (2016) suggests that the effects on a person's physical function and daily activities concluded that there is a "strong correlation" between chronic pain and reduced physical activity. The study also informs us that less than a third of people were able to perform their daily activities due to chronic pain in their back while deterioration was physically noticeable for around 50% of patients who suffer from non-oncological pain. Studies that focus on chronic pain syndrome, such as fibromyalgia, have also reported similar results.

The study by Duenas et al. (2016) also found that chronic pain patients are regularly "unconscious of their level of activity" and patients often report that they are making greater progress than they actually are. It is important that people who suffer from chronic low back pain are aware of their level of activity and maintain their motivation when it comes to becoming more active and living a healthier lifestyle. Otherwise, their condition could worsen before they know it.

Socially, chronic pain can impact the social abilities and interactions of the patient. Such debilitating problems could result in their career being affected, especially if the chronic pain becomes a long-term issue. As Duenas et al. (2016) suggests, people who are suffering from pain may need increased sick leave resulting in decreased productivity. This could deter future promotional or progression opportunities and relationships in the workplace may also suffer, as other colleagues may need to help out more with the tasks you are unable to do. You may also need adaptations, such as an office chair that supports the lumbar area, extra breaks, less time standing or tasks that involve twisting or lifting, and some employees may require shorter working days. If you are unable to fulfil your tasks, the business and other colleagues could suffer too. Over 30% of care-givers are reported to have admitted that they are unable to cope with the pain problems they face and many also included that they suffer with depression and anxiety as a result.

The impact of chronic pain on the person is a world-wide, wide-scale problem that cannot be ignored. That's why it is important to begin to understand the implications of the issues that lower back pain can cause. It influences several aspects of our life, including economical ones. Hence, it is important to build aware-ness about preventing low back problems and the pain that comes with it. There is no doubt that chronic pain creates a domino effect not only as a financial burden but also on the person who suffers from the chronic pain in the lower back area. The question that everyone should be asking right now is - *Will chronic pain go away? And if so, how?* Don't worry, we will cover this soon.

**Will Chronic Pain Go Away?**

First, let's explore the chances of chronic pain subsiding or disappearing. There is a chance that your chronic pain will go away, however, it's important to remember that many chronic pain sufferers deal with the pain for the rest of their lives. Often, this is because they haven't had the opportunity to heal properly or because they have had surgical treatments that require persistent rehabilitation or other treatments to ensure they stay mobile. Many people who have psychological issues also have to deal with the pain for the rest of their lives. Sadly, there is no magic formula to ensure that the pain subsides or disappears indefinitely but there are steps we can take to ensure we keep on-top of our pain issues. Let's look at these now:

**Take Control of Your Pain**

You can do this by ensuring you acknowledge the pain and know how your pain issues affect you. Think about what activities you can still do but acknowledge those you can't. If your pain alters, you should be able to identify this. You should also accept your pain, but this doesn't mean giving up, it means being able to identify your pain and knowing your own body while taking steps to keep in the best possible shape. This is the best way to ensure you receive the most appropriate treatment. You should never reject or ignore pain as this is a negative step that will sabotage your chances of recovery.

## Living Day to Day

Pain can ease or subside some days but return with a vengeance the next. It is important that you recognize the effects of your pain as it builds up. As soon as you begin to recognize these, it will become easier to control them. If you are living with chronic pain, ensure you recognize the effects and respect your limitations. Don't be afraid to allow yourself plenty of recovery time if this is a new injury or pain. Many people don't rest enough, which results in recurring back pain issues.

## Acknowledging Limitations

This is closely linked to the first two steps as it involves taking control and living day-by-day. Accepting your limitations doesn't mean you should stop or give up. It simply means that you should check in with your pain levels and if they're heightened, accept that there are things you may not be able to do that particular day. The main thing here is to ensure you live and enjoy your life. If you feel up to it, do the things you want or have planned to do, but if you're in pain, don't push yourself too hard. Do what you can, but if you're not going to be able to take part in a specific activity, alter your goals. Nothing is set in stone, so stop being so tough on yourself.

## Empowerment

The more you take control and manage your pain, the more empowered you feel. Don't forget to celebrate your wins and your good days but also take advantage of your options. You have the power to choose your path so set small goals and stay motivated in relation to your prescribed treatments.

## Accepting Loss of Self

It is easy to feel loss when you feel there are limitations placed on your life. Don't allow this to be the focus of your day as you are likely to fall into patterns of depression and anxiety. Accept that there are some things you may not be able to do at times but rather than dwelling on it, practice your gratitude. Think about all the things you can do and all the things in your life that you are thankful for. Remember, that's what makes you who you are! Don't forget to ask for help and support if you need it, from health professionals, friends, and family. You are not alone as they are all here for you!

## More to Life than Pain

Although this is a tough one, remember there's more to life than pain. Ensure you don't fall into the chronic pain cycle and focus on your pain as your focus should be on the positives – the things you can do! Try to focus on your strengths and utilize those things to power through. If you are used to going to the gym to lift weights, try going swimming instead as although it's still exercise, it's also a great way to ease pain.

## Don't Fight Battles that Cannot Be Won

There is a popular saying that suggests you should choose your battles wisely and this is a great saying because you should never fight a losing battle. If your body is screaming at you (by sending messages of pain) to rest, take care of your body and rest. Of course, if you have strengthening exercises that you've been told to do, then you should do those (if your healthcare professional instructs) but try not to battle through. Choose your health and wellbeing instead!

## Spiritual Strength

We've talked about meditation a little already but if you really want to improve your chronic pain, you should try becoming spiritual as it can really help improve your state of mind as well as your general health. Things like color therapy, Indian head massage, meditations, tuning forks, and yoga are great ways to develop and grow your spiritual strength. By cleansing your mind, you'll be able to focus clearly on your pain and assess it effectively. This can also strengthen the way you manage your pain as a whole and help you take charge of your recovery.

**ACTIVITY - Recognizing Chronic Pain**

If you want to improve the way you manage your pain, the first step is to recognize your chronic pain. So many people who suffer with pain, do so in silence. Look at the questions below and answer them as honestly as you can.

1. How often does your pain occur?

- a) Every week
- b) Every day
- c) Every month or more

2. How intense is the pain you suffer from? (10 is the worst it could possibly be and 0 is no pain at all.)

- a) 8+
- b) b) 4-8
- c) c) 0-3

3. How often does the pain you suffer from limit your day-to-day activities?

- a) A lot
- b) Little to moderate
- c) Never

4. How are you coping with the pain?

- a) I'm not, it's unbearable
- b) Some days are fine while others are difficult
- c) I cope well with the pain

5. Do you suffer from other symptoms besides the pain (this could include depression, anxiety, another physical or mental health condition, mobility issues, or social issues)?

- a) Yes, all of those
- b) Yes, some of those
- c) No, there are no other symptoms

If you answered *mostly As*, then you are currently suffering from persistent and chronic pain and could possibly have a health condition. Ensure you seek advice from your doctor or other healthcare professional and take action to improve your pain situation.

By following the steps in this book, we can work out the perfect master plan to keep you healthy and focused on remedying your lower back pain.

If you answered *mostly Bs*, then you are suffering from chronic pain but as you feel okay on some days, you are trying to carry on with your life as normal. Seek some advice on how you can maintain your fitness levels and ensure you listen to your body. Rest when you need to but you can make preparations for getting back to normal.

If you answered *mostly Cs*, then you may have very little or no back pain issues right now. That's great news! You should still read this book to increase your awareness about back pain and ensure you follow your maintenance plan. It's important you maintain a healthy lifestyle and still ensure you care for your back to prevent any issues in the future.

## Alternative Ways to Manage Chronic Pain

To close this chapter, it's important that we talk about alternative ways to medical and therapeutic care. If you don't require or want surgery or medication when it comes to healing your chronic back pain, that's great news. There are some alternative therapies out there that you can explore. They include:

1. **Meditation** – We've mentioned this quite a lot so far but it's a great alternative therapy. There are guided meditations out there that focus solely on relieving pain.

2. **Acupuncture** – This alternative therapy can be an amazing experience. Acupuncture originated in China and is able to directly target the painful area.

3. **Hypnotherapy** – If you really don't want to take medication, hypnotherapy can target the cause of your chronic pain issue. For example, if you have poor posture, and it's causing pain, you can use hypnotherapy to target this. It's worth checking out – *what have you got to lose by trying this?*

4. **Deep Breathing Exercises** – There are many different deep breathing exercises that you can use if you want to relax and improve your back health. There are exercises to encourage relaxation, for example, if you sit with your back straight, holding a talk posture, you can breathe in for 5 seconds, hold for 2 seconds, and breathe out for 7 seconds. This can help you relax and focus, so when you breathe out, focus on relaxing the areas that you find painful. If you find this isn't relaxing you, try breathing out for 8 seconds instead. The key is

to breathe out for longer than you breathe in. The holding of the breath should be less than the other two actions.

5. **Biofeedback Options** – To receive biofeedback, you have to undergo a series of noninvasive tests. A medical professional will provide you with the results so that you can make subtle changes to your body in order to reduce pain and improve your health and physical performance. Depending on your health or pain issues, the medical professional may explore your brain wave activity, breathing, heart rate, sweat gland activity, temperature, and muscle contraction. They will then use your results and present you with feedback and advice.

Now that we've explored the burden that chronic pain has on world healthcare and investigated how it impacts a person, we have a broader understanding on the limitations that come with chronic pain and how some people may have better access to healthcare than others. We have also reviewed ways to pinpoint and manage chronic pain and what alternative therapies may be available to us.

Being in persistent pain is not an ideal situation for anyone but rather than ignoring the pain or allowing it to consume us, it is important that we are able to make informed decisions regarding our health and wellbeing. Understanding our pain and taking ownership when it comes to caring for ourselves helps us to continue to live fulfilling, independent, and healthy lives. Simply taking control of the situation can improve our motivation and ensure we do not self-sabotage our recovery.

Back problems are complex, so it's always best to try to get a diagnosis from a health professional, rather than self-diagnosis, but this isn't always a simple matter. In the next chapter, we will focus on getting a diagnosis about low back pain. We will also explore treatment options for all situations, from minor conditions to those that are more severe.

4

INVESTIGATIONS, DIAGNOSIS,
AND TREATMENTS

You must have figured out by now that when it comes to back pain, things are not always a simple or an easy fix. Back pain does not discriminate based on age – you can be young (or young-at-heart) but your back may feel like it's been going for 101 years. The best way forward is to receive a diagnosis, so that you can receive the correct treatment as early as possible. In reality, this often takes time which means that the issue has time to escalate.

In this chapter, we are going to talk through some of the most common back problems from minor to severe conditions and explore what they mean. By the end, we will have considered how they are diagnosed and have explored some traditional diagnostic methods. We will have also looked at possible professional treatments that can improve or cure these conditions.

Building and developing a rounded knowledge and understanding of back problems will increase awareness and help us to prevent further escalated issues. Let's start by introducing diagnosis and treatment, so that you can begin to understand what happens during this process.

**An Introduction to Diagnosis and Treatment**

The best way to receive a diagnosis for your back problem is to visit a medical professional. This should be a qualified practitioner, like a doctor, a chiropractor, or a physiotherapist. At your first consultation, it is likely that the medical professional will ask a series of questions to identify symptoms you are suffering from. This means that they can pinpoint any red flags and check if there are any ominous signs that indicate a particular condition. By reflecting on your patient history, medical professionals can also get a fuller picture and help to rule out certain conditions quite quickly.

Most low back pain stems from the spine and its supporting structure, which includes joint or ligament strain, muscle spasms, or other strains. This type of pain is often labelled as mechanical LBP (low back pain). Your medical professional is likely to request further tests such as X-rays and examine you. Your practitioner will want to discuss pathological findings in the X-ray and the spinal joint functions to check if it affects your mobility, and if so, how. They will also discuss the level of your perceived pain and consider how it is impacting you.

During your physical examination, different orthopedic tests are often used to help identify different possibilities, which can be ruled in or out. Your medical professional is trying to get a deeper understanding of your condition and which structures are affected. This ensures your recovery process to reduce and manage the level of acute pain during this phase. It can help plan which activities should be avoided, initially. Your medical professional should stress the importance of muscle engagement and strength during your recovery period. With this in mind, you should be encouraged during active care to take ownership of your recommended exercises to ensure optimal recovery.

It is important that diagnostic imaging, such as ultrasounds, MRI scans and alike, are not overused when diagnosing low back pain. Even if the imaging shows evidence of pathological findings in the spine, it does not improve the patient's outcome. Once diagnosed, the patient can follow their treatment plan to improve their back health, but it is important to consider what can cause low back in the first place.

**What Can Cause Low Back Pain?**

There are several things that can cause pain in your back. Some are more painful and more serious than others. Let's explore some of these causes:

- **Strain** – This is when the lumbar muscle is strained causing muscles to be torn or stretched in an abnormal way.
- **Sprain** – This is when the ligaments in the lumbar are torn from their attachments.
- **Spondylosis** – This is when the bones and discs in the vertebrae change. This is usually due to intervertebral disc degeneration, osteoarthritis, and stenosis.
- **Intervertebral Disc Degeneration** – This is when the discs in the lumbar region break down and cause pain in your lower back. This can also spread to your neck, legs, and arms.
- **Stenosis** – This is when the spaces between your spine are narrowed. This can compress the nerve and cause pain.
- **Herniated Discs** – This is when the discs between each individual vertebrae are causing you pain due to being damaged because some of

the nucleus is pushing through the annulus. They can put pressure on nerves as a result.

- **Sciatica** – This is a pinching of the nerve roots related to the herniated disc. The pain usually affects the lower back, hip, and thigh. Then, it runs down your outer leg.
- **Piriformis Syndrome** – This is an uncommon neuro-muscular disorder that is similar to sciatica and can mimic its symptoms. The piriformis is a muscle located near the hip joint that can sometimes put pressure on the sciatic nerve.
- **Traumatic Injuries** – This is when injury or pain is caused by an injury, for example, if you were in an accident that hurt your back. This can result in numerous injuries or numbness.
- **Pregnancy** - Low back pain can also be a result of pregnancy. We've touched on this previously, and in many cases, this subsides. It is often down to the way our bodies are changing and a consequence of carrying extra weight.

With some of the more serious conditions, you will need medical investigations. They include:

- **Infections within the Vertebrae** – Although

rare, these are caused by bacteria in the spinal tissues and requires immediate treatment.

- **Intervertebral Discs (Discitis)** – This is usually a bacterial infection between the discs and the vertebrae.

- **Sacroiliac Joint (Sacroiliitis)** - This is inflammation of the sacroiliac joints in the lower spine and pelvis. Pain usually occurs in the lower back or buttocks and can spread to both legs. Climbing or standing for lengthy periods can increase the pain.

- **Cauda Equina Syndrome** – This is a severe type of stenosis. The nerves in the lower back are compressed which causes weakness in both legs. This is a rare condition.

- **Kidney Stones** – They are formed in the kidney but can move into the ureters. Kidney stones can cause low back pain.

- **Severe Osteoporosis** – This is when the bones become increasingly fragile. They are at risk of breaking. This is a health condition common in people who have had trauma injuries.

- **Inflammatory Disease** – This usually happens when blood flow is increased and cells arrive in the area causing pain and swelling. This often results in loss of function too but there is no infection. There isn't always a clear explanation of why this has happened.

- **Endometriosis** – This is a condition that affects the tissue outside the uterus. It can cause pelvic pain and fertility issues. Women who have endometriosis can also suffer from low back pain. This type of pain is often felt deep within the body.

## Diagnostic Methods

There are many ways to diagnose a back problem. First of all, you should speak to a medical professional, so they can arrange for some diagnostic tests to help you get to the root of your back issue.

Diagnostic methods include:

- **X-rays** – to be able to look closely at your bones.
- **MRI** – to look at your bones, joints, blood vessels, and joints.
- **CAT Scan** – a combination of X-rays and computer images to look at your bones and other tissues.
- **Myelography** – an X-ray used alongside contrast dye specially to look for problems in the spinal canal.

- **Lumbar Discography** –an imaging test that looks at the spinal discs and tries to identify any damage which may cause pain or discomfort.
- **Bone Scan** – to closely examine various bones in the skeletal system. This is a specialized radiology procedure that can identify chemical and physical changes within the bones.
- **Blood Tests** –blood is taken and studied to find any markers within your blood work that can indicate what is causing the issues. This can really support your treatment plan.
- **EMG** –measures muscle response or your electrical activity when your nerves are stimulated in a particular area of the body.

Once you've diagnosed the issue, you can begin to consider the treatments available for your particular problem. Next, we will explore some possible treatments that may be available to you.

## Treatments During Acute, Sub-acute, and Chronic Phase

It is important to recognize that treatments are different at each phase. Let's start with the acute phase.

## The Acute Phase

This phase is common when it comes to lower back pain, especially if an injury has been sustained. Serious mechanism injury symptoms can occur if you have been involved in a car crash, a fall from a height, or as a result of heavy lifting when you have underlying osteoporosis. Anyone who has signs of altered sensations, including weakness and numbness, should seek medical attention immediately.

During the acute stage, patients are sometimes suffering from muscle strain or spinal joint sprain and this type of pain usually resolves itself within 2 weeks. Over this time, it is best to use ice treatments to treat your pain symptoms. This is described below:

### *Your Acute Self-Care Routine*

**The First 2 Days:** When using ice, you should always wet a towel and use this as an extra layer between your skin and the ice bag. It can help you to distribute the temperature better and prevent frostbite. You can use tensor bandages to apply further pressure. It is recommended that you use ice treatments twice per day for the first 2 days. You should apply the treatment for 10 minutes followed by 20 minutes of rest.

**From Day 3+:** After 2 days have passed, you can start using heat packs or patches throughout the day. They can help to drastically reduce your painful symptoms and you may start performing your *early recovery routine*. This should consist of stretching and strengthening exercises. We will discuss those in chapters 9 and 10.

If you have not felt any relief from the acute self-care routine above and are still in pain, you should visit a chiropractor, physiotherapist, an athletic therapist, or an osteopath. These four types of health professionals are non-invasive and can assess you and employ different treatment strategies to quickly manage your pain level.

All four types of integrative health professionals can help but you should find someone who is not simply fixated on your pain symptoms. Your health professional should evaluate you as a whole person. This includes looking at your mechanical gait pattern, postural muscle strength through range of motion (ROM) testing, and tightening or contraction of the hip, including the hip musculature with either the anterior or posterior hip tilting. By screening patients, health professionals are able to pick up on mechanical faults which the patient themselves may not even be aware of.

Based on personal and professional experience, along with a combination of spinal adjustments, proprioceptive neuromuscular facilitation (PNF) stretching, soft tissue therapy, electroacupuncture, and a customized exercise routine, improvements can be made to the patient's condition. 95% of patients who come through the door for help consistently report a reduction of pain and notable improvements.

It is important for all sufferers remember that it can take acute pain caused by disc problems 8-12 weeks before they feel pain relief. There is no quick fix – it takes time and perseverance.

## The Sub-acute Phase

As discussed earlier in this book, the sub-acute phase is for those who have conditions or persistent symptoms that last longer than 6 weeks. During this phase, once pain has been minimized, you can become more physically active and incorporate strengthening and stretching exercises.

When the pain is under control, healthcare professional visits usually reduce to once every 2-3 weeks. The meeting includes checking up on their exercise forms and ensuring that these are still intact. As the patient is in control of their own healing process, visits to the clinic are less frequent. In addition, walking is also recommended as the motion encourages nutrients to flow around the body and pump into your discs while increasing the circulation around the body. This can increase healing.

If a patient is suffering from spinal or central stenosis, using a stationary exercise bike can help lessen disc pressure. Proprioceptive exercises and visiting either a physical therapist or chiropractor who emphasize the importance of stretching exercises can really help with your rehabilitation. When exercising to rehabilitate following low back pain, ensure you receive proper guidance. In addition to this, you can speak to your health professional. There are some excellent examples available on YouTube but always ensure you are following a professional physical therapist or chiropractor (any legitimate practitioner will gladly provide links to their websites, so you can check them out). Poor exercise guidance can lead to further issues, so don't take any risks!

If your pain persists over a longer period of time, then your healthcare professional should write to your physician. This is something that usually happens between 8-10 weeks and it gives your healthcare professional the opportunity to work in collaboration with your physician. This usually results in the patient being referred for epidural or cortisone injections but this should be a last resort as it isn't solving the problem. It is simply numbing the pain temporarily. This isn't something that I would personally want for my patients.

When a patient can finally move 80% and above for ranges in motion, they can start to complete exercises to strengthen the lower back. *How to Strengthen the Lower Back* on Medical News Today provides 10 great exercises to help you strengthen your core muscles and prevent low back pain.

## Chronic Pain

If you are suffering from chronic pain in the lower back area, you should always see a healthcare or medical professional. They can get to the root of the problem and provide advice and guidance. You should never take action until you have been advised by a professional when it comes to chronic pain. The best course of action in the meantime is to rest and take pain relief if necessary.

Pain is something that we can't control but must learn to manage. While we can't choose the pain, we can choose our healthcare professional and treatment options.

## Treatment Options

Choosing your treatment is something you should consider carefully. Remember, you should always choose to see a healthcare or medical professional first, but other treatment options may be an option.

Complementary therapies concentrate on calming your body and mind. They reduce stress and encourage you to relax while relieving anxiety. They can help you improve your general health and well-being and they can even calm your emotions and create a more positive mindset. This helps you feel good!

There are a number of available treatments that can be beneficial when it comes to low back pain. Be sure to seek advice from your medical or healthcare professional first, as they can consider your condition and treatment phase before recommending alternative complementary or holistic therapies. Alternative methods are certainly worth considering when you're recovering and are great self-care opportunities.

Numerous complementary therapies that may be beneficial to you. These include:

- **Chiropractic** – This is when your chiropractor uses their hands to adjust the joints of the spine and work on muscles and ligaments to relieve problems in that particular area. In addition, chiropractor will include exercises to facilitate the rehabilitation process.
- **Physical Therapy** – This is when a physical

therapist uses massage, exercise, and heat treatments to treat your pain or injury rather than surgery or drugs.

- **Acupuncture and Electro-acupuncture** – Acupuncture is an ancient Chinese complementary therapy in which fine needles are inserted into the skin at specific pressure points. This is used for both physical and mental conditions.
- **Massage Therapy** – This is when massage is used to alleviate pain and anxiety for people who have several conditions, including back pain.
- **Yoga** – This is a form of gentle exercise that focuses on flexibility, strength, and breathing. It can help to strengthen the muscles and is known for helping you maintain healthy joints and a healthy back.
- **Aqua Therapy** – Sometimes, this is referred to as hydrotherapy. This is when activities, such as light exercises, are performed in water. This can help in rehabilitation and recovery situations when injuries have occurred.
- **Inversion Table** – This is sometimes referred to as spinal traction. Basically, this involves being turned upside down whilst on a special table. It is said that gravity eases the pressure

you feel on your discs and nerves. It is also a
great way to gently stretch muscles and joints
and can be very relaxing. However, inversion
therapy does not provide lasting relief and is
not safe for everyone. By remaining in an
inverted position, heart beats can slow down
causing increased blood pressure and the
pressure within the eyeballs can increase
drastically. If you have high blood pressure,
heart disease, or glaucoma, you should not try
inversion therapy

We've discussed non-invasive, complementary therapies that may be used when you're in recovery but
sometimes those are not enough. Although medication
should only be used if it's absolutely necessary, pain can
be debilitating and therefore, it is important to consider
over-the-counter medications that you may use for
lower back pain.

**Over-the-counter Remedies**

When it comes to back pain, we shouldn't dismiss the
fact that sometimes over-the-counter remedies may be
beneficial, especially if your pain is affecting your daily
life. The problem with medication is that it can lead to
drug overdoses. People can also become addicted to
pain relief medication. According to the National Insti-

tute on Drug Abuse, almost 50,000 people died in the US from opioid drug overdoses. This is because they are overprescribed to patients and many are readily available to buy over the counter. Always consider your other options before you revert to pain medication. They should only be used if absolutely necessary.

NSAIDs are also widely used to reduce inflammation and relieve pain, especially if the sufferer is a long-term pain sufferer. NSAID stands for Non-Steroidal Anti-Inflammatory Drugs. You can use these instead of opioid drugs and although you can take these orally, you can also get them in patch form for slow release. Some pain-relief creams which you rub into the painful area can also contain NSAIDs.

The most common medications prescribed for low back pain by a doctor are benzodiazepines and diclofenac. When it comes to medication, it is always advised that you discuss your options with a medical professional. Ask your doctor for more information on suitable medications you can use to treat your pain and don't be afraid to ask questions if you have any concerns.

**Surgical Considerations**

Sometimes, it is impossible to ignore surgical procedures as an option to cure or improve low back pain.

Let's quickly explore these, and that way, if your medical or healthcare professional suggests any of these things, you know what they are.

- **Trigger Point Injection** – This is a procedure involving an injection that treats the muscle trigger points, which are the contracted knots or spasms that you can feel under your skin.
- **Guided Epidural** – This is a steroid injection performance at a doctor's office. It can help to target the painful area and numb the pain.
- **Facet Injections** – The target area will be X-rayed and numbed, and then steroids are injected in. The facet joints link the bones in your spine together. After the injections, you generally need two days to recover.
- **Radiofrequency Denervation** – This is a treatment for back pain that comes from your facet joints. Again, this means a needle is inserted into the damaged joint. Typically, a local anesthetic numbs the nerve first before you receive the injections.

## Medical Emergencies

Sometimes, a back injury or back pain can become an emergency and surgical intervention is required. If your healthcare professional thinks surgery is a suitable option for you, they may consider one of the following surgical procedures:

- **Discectomy** – This is when the damaged portion of your herniated disc has to be removed via a surgical procedure.
- **Lumbar Fusion** – This is typically recommended when you need to stop the painful vertebral segment from its painful, abnormal motion. This often involves adding a bone graft to a segment of the spine.
- **Disc Replacement** – This is when a disc is replaced by an artificial disc in the lumbar area.

Now that we've looked at low back pain diagnosis as well as the different treatments available, it is time to change our habits to improve our back care for good. If you're ready to work on how to consistently maintain a healthy back, you are certainly ready to move onto the next chapter.

# 5

# A HEALTHY BACK = A HAPPIER YOU

It's quite simple. If you want a healthy back, then you must take care of it and part of taking care of your back includes developing healthy back habits. Having good habits in relation to your back can prevent issues from recurring and improve the general health of your back, even strengthening it so you are less likely to suffer from such injuries. Having a habit means you repeatedly do something without thinking about it. For example, we automatically wash our hands before we handle food (or at least we should) and this is a habit because we do it so often that it becomes second nature to us. Having healthy back habits means you'll constantly, but naturally, take measures that ensure you prevent and maintain a healthy back!

In this chapter, we will talk about maintaining a healthy back. We will also discuss the fundamentals of your daily activities and review the mechanics involved in those. Nobody is excluded from this chapter – daily back habits are for *everyone*. This includes people who already have lower back pain and those who don't but want to take preventative measures. We will discuss the benefits of having an exercise routine, which includes stretching, and talk about how this can decrease your chance of low back pain attacks. When it comes to back pain, movement is often medicine as it ensures we maintain good posture. Now let's start with what you need to look out for before you begin!

**What If I Have Symptoms or Pain Already?**

Before you begin, you should assess yourself. To assess yourself, follow the steps below:

- Go somewhere quiet where you will not be disturbed.
- Close your eyes.
- Breathe in for 5 seconds, hold for 2 seconds, and then breathe out for 7 seconds. Repeat a few times until you begin to feel relaxed.
- Think about the following questions:

1. How do I feel?
2. Can I feel tension in any part of my body?
3. Does anywhere hurt?

- Then, begin with your head and work your way down, scanning every part of your body. Some people prefer to do this with their eyes closed still, which is fine.
- Take your time and visualize each part of your body from head to toe thinking about how each part feels. *What do you notice?*

If you notice any parts of your body that have tension or any pain, you really need to be careful when it comes to exercise – they will need to be considered. While some exercises will help pain, it is important to ensure that you don't compromise any other parts of your body in the meantime. It is also important to watch out for any radicular symptoms that could prevent or limit our exercise regime before you begin. This includes numbness or altered sensations that may travel down the legs. Another symptom could include weakness. In relation to exercise, it is important that you seek medical attention before you embark or pursue any exercise routine.

## How Habits Are Formed

We've mentioned habits previously. These are the things we do naturally without really thinking about them. Nobody reminds us that we have to put one foot in front of the other when walking, and that's because we've done this so many times, we do it automatically without thinking.

If you want to create good habits, you need to consistently repeat an activity over and over again. Practice, practice, practice! Essentially, you are making the habit a part of your routine, and eventually, you'll do this automatically without thinking.

When my patients are considering a stretching routine, many complain that they do not have enough time but forming habits takes time and it's important that you make time for this. By taking time, you are:

- Saving yourself time in the future because if you allow your back pain to escalate, it will take more time to fix later.
- Taking care of yourself, which makes you start to feel valued as a person.
- Allowing yourself to feel good. If you stretch off your back, it can make you feel good, and anyone who feels good generally performs

better when completing daily tasks and activities.

Only you can decide to allocate the time to yourself. Really consider what's more important when you take a "break". *Would you rather watch Netflix or scroll through your phone, or will you take some time to take care of yourself and your health?* By taking just 10 minutes from your regular, leisurely activities to stretch and strengthen your muscles, you can make a vast improvement to your health.

**Improving Posture**

Stretching and strengthening your muscles can help you improve your posture. Bad posture can cause a long list of back problems, so looking after it can help you maintain a healthy back. If you spend a lot of time working on a computer or sitting down at a desk, posture issues are common. By building an awareness of your posture, you can improve that easily.

Poor posture can lead to tension headaches, imbalance, and several types of aches and pains. It puts pressure on the integrity of our back muscles, ligaments, tendons, and discs. The pain can worsen and lead to further issues if you don't take action, and therefore, it is important to maintain good posture and be aware of any persisting problems.

To keep good posture, you should:

- Sit or stand up tall and straight.
- Roll back your shoulders.
- Keep your stomach pulled in.
- Keep your head level.
- When standing, keep your feet shoulder-width apart and let your arms hang loosely.

This is your natural good posture, so pay attention to how that feels and you will begin to recognize when you are starting to stray. Maintaining good posture is the best possible way to support your spine and maintain good back health.

**Stretching Components**

Stretching your lower back has many positive benefits. First of all, it improves your flexibility as well as your range of motion. Flexibility is important if you want to be able to perform everyday activities and it can generally improve your mobility. Having a good motion range provides you with the ability to move freely when twisting, turning, and bending. If you follow a stretching regime, it can actually increase your range of motion. As many people with low back issues begin to notice limitations in relation to their flexibility and motion, stretching can help prevent or overcome such issues.

Stretching also increases the blood flow to your muscles as doing this on a regular basis is said to improve your circulation. As a result of increased circulation, you may find that your injury recovery period is shortened, especially when you are subject to muscle soreness. Generally, stretching improves your performance when it comes to physical activities too, especially if you do your stretches before you take part in a specific activity.

Stretching the muscles in your lower back can also help to prevent back pain. If you already suffer from low back pain, it can help to heal this too. That's because stretching the muscles in your back can aid recovery. In addition, it also reduces stress and improves your posture. As previously mentioned, back pain can increase tension headaches, and therefore, stretching can help to reduce the chance of those while also calming your mind. The one question that come from patients at this stage is: *what stretches should I be doing?*

You should consider the common forms of stretching, which are dynamic and static. Dynamic stretches are usually carried out to prepare you for movement. They cause your muscles to stretch, and although they are active movements, the stretch is not held in the end position. In comparison, static stretches are used after you exercise and involve holding the stretch. You don't have to hold the stretch for a long time – it is usually between 10-30 seconds. You can incorporate these into your 10-minute regime.

Remember, you should stay safe when exercising, so, you SHOULDN'T:

- **Overdo It** – Take it easy and ensure you don't overstretch.
- **Bounce** – It can cause an injury due to the impact on the body.
- **Push Your Stretch to a Feeling of Discomfort** – don't make the pain worse, simply back off until the stretch is more comfortable.
- **Go into Your Stretches Cold** – Warm up a little by walking for 5-10 minutes beforehand.

Here are seven exercises to help improve low back pain and your posture:

## 1. The Upper Body and Arm Stretch

To do this, you should be seated in a chair with your back straight. Put your arms above your head and clasp your hands together with your hands facing up. Push your arms up and stretch your whole body upwards.

Hold the stretch for 10 seconds and then release. Do this 5 times.

## 2. Torso Stretch

To do this, stay seated but shuffle towards the front of the chair. Cross your right leg over the other and place your right arm on the back of the chair. Place your left hand on your left knee and gently twist your neck and body to look over your right shoulder. Hold for 10 seconds, then slowly move into a forward-facing position. Repeat this three times, and then repeat on the other side too.

## 3. Hip and Knee Stretch

To do this, lean back in the chair and put both feet on the floor. Pull one knee towards your chest and hug it. Hold for 10 seconds and then release. Alternate with your other leg. You should do this 5 times on each side.

## 4. The Cat or Cow Stretch

To do this, you should kneel on the floor on all fours. Ensure your hands are positioned below your shoulders. Your knees should also be in line with your hips. As you exhale, you should gently arch your spine and hold for 3 seconds. Then, inhale and round off your back. Be sure to tighten your core muscles and hold this for 3 seconds. Do this 5 times.

## 5. Half Cobra Pose

To do this, you should lay flat on the floor, on your front. Put your forehead onto the floor and put your hands at the sides of your face, just above your shoulders. Push up from the floor, raising your head so you are facing forward and arching your back. Hold for 10-15 seconds, then lower back down and repeat. Do this 5 times.

## 6. Shoulder Raises

Raise both shoulders up towards the ears and then drop them. Repeat this 10 times. You can also incorporate a roll here by raising the shoulders and rolling them forwards on the drop. You can also roll them back. If you do this, ensure you roll them forwards 10 times, and then repeat, rolling them back 10 times.

## 7. Upper Trap Stretch

To do this, you should raise your right arm and place it over your head, so it's reaching the left side. Gently pull your head towards your right shoulder until you feel a light stretch. Hold your pose for 10-15 seconds. Repeat this 3 times and then repeat this on the other side too.

The exercise routine above should get you started on the right track when it comes to your own healthy back regime. Now, let's focus on strengthening your muscles.

**Strengthening Component**

It is important to ensure the muscles in your lower back are kept strong. Strength in the back is not necessarily more muscle mass. It is about activation of the muscles and neuromuscular stabilization. Core strength and glute strength is important as it can help with balance.

In clinical practice, we perform strength tests for all lower limb muscles that govern hip movements. Imbalances are often present in the majority of acute to chronic low back pain sufferers. Strength testing is an important component when treating such issues.

There are many exercises that can assist you in strengthening your lower back. It is important to remember that you should get medical advice before you complete an exercise routine. Let's look at four low impact exercises that will help to strengthen your lower back muscles. You may wish to incorporate them into your routine as they will ensure a healthy back.

**1. Glute Bridge**

Lay on your back with your hands down by your side. Bend your knees and ensure your feet are flat to the floor. Push your stomach into the air raising your bottom off the ground. When you're resting only on your shoulder blades, arms, and feet, hold for 20 seconds and then lower the back down to the floor again, slowly. Repeat 5 times.

## 2. The Plank

Lie on your stomach with your forearms flat to the ground. Lift your body, so you are solely resting on your toes and forearms. Keep your back straight and don't raise your bottom too high. Everything should be as straight as possible. Hold this position for 30 seconds and aim to repeat this 2-3 times. If this is too demanding, please put your knees down onto the ground for support, instead of using just your toes. You can then build up to the plank over time with practice.

## 3. Leg Raises

Lay down on the floor on your stomach. Place your palms under your forehand. Straighten one leg and then lift it a few inches off the ground. Hold for 3 seconds and bring it down. Repeat 10 times. Remember to switch legs and do the other side too.

## 4. Lower Trunk Rotation

Lay down on your back with your knees bent and your feet elevated so that it appears as if you're sitting on a chair from a lying position. Place your arms out to the sides at shoulder height and hold them steady. Keep your knees together and slowly, lower your knees to one side towards the floor. Make sure you constantly steady yourself. Hold for 3 seconds and take a deep breath before rolling them back up to the center. Repeat on the other side. You should do at least 3 of these on each side.

Remember, these exercises can help you to strengthen your muscles, tendons, and ligaments, which can result in a healthier back. You should choose the exercises that work for you and it is important to listen to your body – no exercise should ever cause you pain. It is always a good idea to start small. So, in the beginning, start off with just doing one of each of the four strengthening exercises listed above. You can build them up over time. Listening to your body is the key to maintaining a healthy back!

## Cardio Component

We've mentioned cardio already and discussed the importance of warming up before you start an exercise routine. You should always do this before you start your strengthening and stretching exercises as it prepares your body for movement.

Cardio exercise is great for low back pain. That's because such aerobic activity helps the blood flow around your body, feeding the brain and your muscles. This means that the nutrients in your soft tissues, which you need to heal your back issues, arrive at the painful area much quicker. Your back issues are therefore resolved because your muscles have everything they need to repair themselves swiftly. However, this doesn't mean cardio is always easy for those with low back pain.

Even though it can be beneficial, you need to be really careful with this type of exercise when you are suffering from pain symptoms as you don't want to make things worse. It is best to do a short bout of cardiovascular activity and build it up gradually. Start with 5 minutes, and over time, build this up to 20-30 minutes. It is believed that altering blood flow in the different regions of the brain for acute and chronic lower back pain patients can lead to unconscious pain behavior.

Great examples of cardio exercise includes:

- Walking
- Running
- Jogging
- Skipping
- Squats
- Swimming
- Burpees
- Jumping Jacks

When you are considering cardio exercise, always consider what you can or can't do right now. For example, starting with a short walk is great to begin with, but then you may walk for longer and even start jogging. Eventually, you may start running, again starting with a short run, and then building up to a longer run.

When it comes to exercise routines, everyone is different. Many people aggravate their injuries because they don't listen to their bodies. We all have limitations and it's important that we recognize these. Take it slow!

**Body Mechanics**

When we lay in a specific position or constantly repeat the same movements, we can become stiff or suffer from ligament creeps. As a result, our muscles are delayed or react to this mechanical load. It is important that we remember this when we consider maintaining a healthy back. Let's look at some occasions when our body mechanics may be affected:

## Sleep

Sleep is really important if you want to maintain a healthy back. Your spine needs a good night's rest and it deserves to be nurtured. But, *did you know that some sleeping positions can actually cause you pain?* Let's look at some sleeping tips and tricks to help you lessen low back pain and acute pain.

## Your Bed

Let's start with your bed. You should have a healthy mattress if possible as this is the key to ensuring you are comfortable. Mattresses are not cheap and it is important to ensure that it is not too soft nor too hard. Your mattress needs to be good for you and your condition, so if you have a recurring back injury, speak to your healthcare professional for advice.

## Climbing in and out of Your Bed

Climbing into your bed can actually cause you discomfort if you are suffering from pain. The best thing to do is to carefully perch on the edge of your bed and use your arms to lower your torso while bringing up your legs. You can then roll onto your back, but you should avoid twisting. You should try to keep your hips in line while doing this. When doing this, you can repeat this motion in reverse order by rolling onto your side and sliding your legs off the bed carefully. If you keep the muscles in your abdomen tight and use your hand and elbow to push into the mattress, you should comfortably make it back into your initial seating position.

## Sleeping on Your Stomach

This particular sleeping position can put pressure on your back and neck, so this is not recommended if you are trying to combat low back pain.

## Sleeping on Your Side

To get into this sleeping position, you need to keep your neck and hips in alignment. You can do this by climbing into bed as instructed above and rolling onto your side ensuring you have a medium-sized pillow under your head. Your head and body should be raised equally. If you suffer from low back pain, you could support the arch of your neck by placing a small cushion or towel roll. It is also a good idea to place a thin pillow between your knees as this helps to support your lower back.

## Sleeping on Your Back

When you climb into bed as instructed above, you will be typically lying on your back, but it's important to learn the correct position to lie in if you want to prevent low back pain. The 'supine' position helps ensure that you do not put undue stress on parts of your spine. Once you're in bed, you should use a medium-sized pillow under your head. This means your head and body are equally raised. You can then place a small pillow under the arch of your lower back, as this will give extra support to your spine. You can also place a pillow (or two if needed) under your knees. This helps to keep your spine in a supported, neutral position.

Sleep is an important element when it comes to low back pain as rest is so important for you and your body. Ensuring you get into bed and sleep in the correct way, can help you maintain a healthy back.

## Workstation

Many people work from a workstation when at work as they may be required to use a computer regularly. This can lead to many aches and pains. There are four key areas that you should consider when setting up your workstation.

This includes:

### 1. Your Head Position

Your head is actually a heavy object which is supported by your spine. If you don't sit in the correct position, your head can put more pressure on the spine. Sitting in a neutral position is best as the further away your head is from your spine, the heavier it feels to your spine. Focus on your head being in line with your spine and place your computer screen straight in front of you. Ensure it's positioned within your eye line by propping it up to the right level.

## 2. Your Arm Position

The preferred position for your arms when you're sitting or standing is 90 degrees. This means that your shoulders should be down and relaxed while your elbows should be bent. Your wrists should stay in a neutral position in front of you. Try to keep them loose.

## 3. Your Back

When it comes to your back position, you should start with the feet. Ensure your feet are flat to the floor and your legs and thighs should be parallel with your seat cushion. This may mean you have to lower your seat but this is the correct way to sit in your chair. Your feet should never be propped up or hanging loosely. Keep your back as straight as possible by pushing it up against the back of your chair. While we tend to move forward and backward from time to time, maintain your awareness and ensure you push back into the correct position. If you are uncomfortable, try using a lumbar cushion in the arch of your back. Ensure that your head is over your neck and shoulders at all times and lean your shoulders back against the back of the chair. If your tailbone is causing you pain, you can get cushions which have a piece removed for your tailbone.

It is worth looking into this if you suffer from discomfort here.

## 4. Your Movement

If we sit in the same position for a long period of time, it can cause us pain. We can become stiff, especially if we keep repeating the same movement over and over, day after day. Our joints naturally oil themselves when we move which prevents stiffness, so movement prevents this from happening. The best way to avoid discomfort is to set a reminder in your schedule that reminds you to move. You can simply complete a single stretch, walk to the kitchen to make a refreshment, or even stand up while on a call and roll your shoulders or hips. Ensure you take advantage of your break times and lunch times by going on a short walk. Some people even have the advantage of a sitting and standing desk and are able to alternate throughout the day.

These tips and tricks can prevent low back pain at your workstation but when it comes to household chores, there are more tips and tricks to consider. Let's look at those next.

## Doing Household Chores

Now the household chores need to be done but we can try to do them in the best way that ensures we remain pain free. Let's look at three common household tasks and discuss how we can complete them without over-doing it and causing any further low back pain:

- **Laundry** – If you suffer from low back pain, you should avoid doing the laundry on a low surface. This creates an unfavorable position for your lower back and can lead to further issues, including ligament creeps. Try working on higher surfaces above your waste but below your chest as this will be much more comfortable for you.

- **Washing the Dishes** – If you are constantly washing dishes, you should maintain good posture. By maintaining an upright position, your back will be much more supported, but if you lean forward or bend, it can cause discomfort. Try to squat low rather than leaning or bending but remember to keep your back as straight as possible. This isn't always the easiest way to get lower, but it will help you avoid neck pain and back pain.

- **Vacuuming** – When vacuuming, you are pushing the item forward and then dragging it back. This movement can cause repeated movements that overwork your back. If you want to maintain a healthy back but want to avoid straining yourself, keep your hips and shoulders moving towards the way you are working. Try your best not to bend and stay as upright as possible, but when stretching out over, try lunging forward rather than bending. You can now purchase lighter vacuums, which are great for people who suffer with low back pain as they put less strain on your spine.

You can use the above tips and tricks when completing other household chores too. For example, instead of vacuuming, you can use the same principle for mopping the floor or raking the garden. If you use these tips and tricks and build them into your household chores routine, this way of your body to protect your back will become a habit.

**Nursing Baby**

It is important to consider the impact that breast-feeding can have on you if you have low back issues. The best thing to do if you are nursing your baby is to become aware of your body and discover positions where your body feels balanced. For instance, many women find it more comfortable to be seated and use cushions for support. Cushions can be used to prop up your arm underneath the baby and they can also support the lumbar area. You can buy special pillows such as nursing pillows and neck pillows to support this. You can even buy lumbar pillows. When feeding your baby, you should sit up as straight as possible and maintain good posture, but try to avoid tension as it's important you feel comfortable and relaxed too.

You should start in a typical position that supports your low back. Hold your head above your spine in a neutral position, as we discussed earlier, and ensure your ribcage is aligned with your pelvis. Your pelvis should also be in line with your feet, so you can comfortably remain upright. When in this position, really tune into your body and consider where you need support. Make your own adjustments and then check in with yourself again. *Is this an improvement?* Start moving slightly to compensate for any imbalances, compressions, and twists.

When nursing, you may also need to provide extra support to your breasts. They will be carrying extra weight, so ensure you wear a good bra or shoulder girdle. You should also consider exercising your upper back muscles to strengthen them.

Remember, you don't have to stay still when feeding – you can move around if it's comfortable to do so. You can also do some stretches as soon as you've finished nursing to help loosen up your muscles. Try rolling your shoulders forward and backwards or bring your arms over your head to stretch your upper back and shoulders.

## Pregnancy

We've mentioned pregnancy already, and as you know, low back pain is common in pregnancy. There are some ways in which you can avoid this becoming a problem. Here are some things you can do to avoid back pain throughout your pregnancy:

- Avoid lifting heavy objects, as you shouldn't be doing this anyway.
- Bend with your knees when you pick something up or lift something from a low surface but try to keep your back straight.
- Wear flat shoes as it will help you distribute your weight evenly.
- If you feel pain, take a warm bath or get a massage.
- Avoid twisting. You can simply shuffle or turn by moving your feet.
- Ensure you're supporting your spine when in bed. Put a pillow between your knees, a pillow under your lumbar area, or use maternity support pillows.
- Try to get plenty of rest. Remember, you're

carrying extra weight and it's a strain on your body, so it needs rest to recover.

- If you're carrying your groceries, try to distribute the weight easily (1 bag of the same or similar weight in each hand, for instance) to balance yourself out.

## Weight and Nutrition

We all know that extra weight and obesity can cause low back pain. So many people have an unhealthy weight level these days, and it is important that everyone understands the way this can impact your body. Low back pain is more common in overweight patients than it is in patients who maintain a healthy weight. Sometimes, by simply losing a few pounds, we can remedy our low back issues.

If a person is overweight, their spinal structures, discs, and muscles are often strained. In severe cases, it can result in a pinched nerve, a herniated disc, or sciatica. If you lose weight, it can decrease the risk of you developing any other back problems too, especially if you manage your weight loss through diet, exercise, and nutrition. This can also reduce your pain.

When considering weight loss as a way to remedy your back issue, you should do this in a safe way. You can develop your own safe weight loss diet and exercise program, but you should always speak to your health professional first as they will provide you with the best advice on how to move forward. All diets should be balanced to receive the recommended amount of nutrients and vitamins into your system. You need them to heal and recover following a back injury or back pain symptoms in a reliable, safe, and healthy way. As discussed earlier in this chapter, exercises can help you strengthen and stretch the muscles you need to maintain a healthy back.

Now that you understand the fundamentals of your daily activities and the mechanics involved in maintaining a healthy back, you'll understand that maintaining a healthy back and healthy back habits are for everyone – even busy moms!

We've begun to discuss nutrition in this chapter, but in order to understand its true power when it comes to maintaining a healthy back, read on as we'll focus on this in the next chapter.

# 6

# A DYNAMIC DIET - HOW TO USE NUTRITION TO CONTROL PAIN

Although we've touched on nutrition already, this topic deserves a chapter on its own. That's because nutrition is extremely important if you want to remedy or prevent back injury, and in this chapter, we're going to learn how this can happen. By the end, you'll understand just how important this is!

Nutrition helps our muscles, ligaments, and tendons to heal, for instance, some nutrients have anti-inflammatory properties which can reduce swelling and the pain that goes along with it. With that in mind, we'll provide guidance and tips to ensure your daily nutritional habits lead to optimal body health. This means it keeps us pain free!

## Introduction to a Healthy Diet and Weight Management

Before we go any further, let's consider the pain you feel and how weight can impact this. Around 30% of patients who come through the door in clinics have no obvious cause of pain. This means that they have suffered from no trauma or falls but they begin feeling pain. They don't know why they feel pain and therefore it's not easy to fix it.

Let's consider this patient profile:

- Michael is 35 years old and he weighs 350lbs.
- He woke up with back pain one day and now suffers with chronic pain.
- He also suffers regularly with joint soreness, so if he stands from a sitting position, his breath is taken.

A clinician should always address their patient's weight and diet, especially if they believe it could be contributing to pain and joint soreness. Following this, they should then go over the patient's nutritional regime and help them to modify their diet – replace certain fats with healthy fats and increase the intake of fruit and vegetables while decreasing processed goods. The impact of this can be assessed after 3 months. If the patient has started to lose weight and their energy levels have increased, it means that the patient is on the right track in relation to their diet, especially if the patient has less episodes of joint pain attacks.

Other clients may try other diets such as the Keto Diet, and while there are tremendous results when it comes to weight loss, it is not sustainable in the long term.

While many patients know that nutrition is important, some need simplified visualization and a breakdown of how to put together a healthy meal on their plate. Going through it often helps everyone to gain a stronger understanding of how to choose food wisely. It is thought that 1 in 10 adults do not meet the dietary guideline of minimum intake when it comes to fruits and vegetables. Americans are generally over ingesting sugars, fats, sodium, and sweeteners instead.

Rather than focusing on a more balanced diet and the amount of fruit and vegetables that provide our bodies with the nutrients it needs, the standard American Diet focuses on calorie intake. This can often be the wrong approach as we should be focusing on reducing added fats and sweeteners while increasing our intake of fruits and vegetables.

*So, what's the truth about dieting?*

It is knowing that everything should be in moderation. For example, too much red or processed meat could cause heart disease, stroke, and type 2 diabetes. Red meat is also much more difficult for the digestive system to digest, and therefore, its inability to move means a shorter life expectancy. By incorporating some replacements into your diet, you can change that. You could lower animal-based proteins with non-animal-based proteins such as tofu, quinoa, and legumes.

## What Are 'Whole Foods'?

Whole foods are those that are natural and not processed. They are healthier for you as they do not have manufactured ingredients such as added starches, sugars, and flavorings. Since whole foods are natural, they are an important part of a healthy diet as they contain many nutrients. They usually contain fiber, minerals, and vitamins. Many people who tend to eat a lot of whole foods as part of their diets often claim to be 'eating clean'.

Whole foods are a way of living rather than simply being a temporary diet. The foods are non-addictive, but because they are healthy, the people who follow this often have much more energy and are less likely to be overweight as the foods are much lower in fat.

The basic concept of whole foods is to eat natural foods in the healthiest way. For example, you may eat boiled potatoes instead of potato chips, or instead of fried chicken nuggets, you may eat grilled chicken breast. The best way to check whether the food you are buying is whole food is by reading the labels and checking out what the food contains, including the fat content. Typically, grains, fruit, vegetables, nuts, and beans, along with some meat and cheese are whole. Ready meals and ready-to-eat foods are often not whole as they contain a high content of fat, sodium, or sugar (or sometimes all 3). When it comes to meat, it is sometimes best to buy organic as this signifies that your food is natural. You should also avoid canned foods – things like canned beans are not a whole food.

Fish, dark, leafy greens, legumes, and whole grains are often the best types of whole foods along with eggs and other dairy products. Healthy fats in the likes of olive oil, walnuts, and avocados are also okay to eat too. As we said at the beginning of this chapter – everything in moderation!

**Inflammation and the Immune System**

There is nothing simple about stress and the immune system – it's complicated but let's look at this for a moment. Our bodies are sensitive to stress but there are different types of stress – it is an adaptable energy.

We have good psychological stress when we're feeling energized as we know we are going to be put under mental pressure, like when we're taking an exam for instance. We can also have good physical stress, like the type we experience on our muscles when we're exercising. Maybe you've heard the saying, "feel the burn!", which is typically said when someone is having a good workout. Sometimes, our stress becomes more severe, and this can have a detrimental impact on our health. Unhealthy stress could include us not recovering from mental, emotional, or physical stress appropriately. This could be as a result of injury, depression, or worrying thoughts. If we are suffering from feelings of stress over a lengthy period, the body begins to release increased levels of cortisol. This is used to regulate our immune system and our inflammatory responses because our tissues are sensitive to this. If we suffer from prolonged psychological and chronic stress, the body is unable to regulate itself in the right way. Increased levels of psychological stress leads to chronic inflammation. The inflammation is beneficial but constant tissue breakdown caused through inflammation can weaken our immune system. This means you are likely to suffer from continual infections.

There are some whole foods that can help boost our immune system and have anti-inflammatory properties. This includes things like blueberries, ginger, green tea, and dark chocolate.

Chronic inflammation can cause you a high level of pain. You can combat this by following a healthy diet that focuses on whole foods, and avoids saturated fats, trans-fats, and refined sugars. Risks of chronic pain are even higher for those who are overweight or suffer from diabetes. Other risks include obesity, smoking, age, and both stress and sleep disorders. These things slow down the healing process.

Some of the symptoms of chronic inflammation include body pain, fatigue, insomnia, mood disorders such as depression and anxiety, stomach issues, and weight issues (gain or loss). If you constantly find yourself suffering from infections, this can also be a symptom. Sadly, there are no direct tests that can confirm chronic inflammation. Diagnosis is generally made when the inflammation occurs. There are some blood tests that can indicate chronic inflammation markers, and there is also a serum protein electrophoresis which can also check for markers. Ultimately, chronic inflammation is a complex thing and can be difficult to diagnose.

The best way to treat or manage chronic inflammation is through diet and exercise. You can do this by having a low-glycemic diet, reducing your intake of trans and saturated fats, and increasing your intake of whole foods which we've discussed in the previous section. Things like fish oils, curcumin, and mung beans have strong anti-inflammatory properties. In the previous chapter, we discussed the benefits of physical exercise which is also a great way to combat chronic inflammation.

There are some medications that can be prescribed for chronic pain but this should only be used as a last resort. This is something you can discuss with your medical professional once all other avenues have been explored.

**Plant Based Diet vs Animals Incorporated Diet**

Many people consider a plant-based diet as opposed to an animal-based diet because there are many health benefits. Plant-based diets are becoming increasingly popular due to their varying benefits. They are great if you want to stay healthy and are certainly worth considering. A plant-based diet focuses on naturally grown foods and the person generally avoids animal products. Plant-based doesn't necessarily mean the same as vegan. A vegan person is committed to avoiding meat and does not eat it at all as part of their diet. A person who is on a plant-based diet may occasionally eat meat, fish, and dairy products but their main focus is whole foods that are healthy rather than anything that is processed.

The benefits of a plant-based diet include:

1. Better weight management.
2. Lower risks of underlying health conditions such as heart disease, stroke, high cholesterol, strokes, and high blood pressure.
3. Better general health and increased energy levels.

**An Anti-Inflammatory Diet for Back Pain**

If you're a back pain sufferer looking for a healthy way to keep on top of your condition, you should consider the Flexitarian Diet. This diet focuses mostly on plant-based products but it allows animal products in moderation. The diet incorporates a small amount of red meat and encourages more fish protein.

The health benefits of a Flexitarian diet include a decreased risk of diabetes, a reduced risk of heart disease, and weight loss when required. It has also been linked to cancer and is said to be a positive preventative measure. As you are reducing your meat consumption, this diet is good for the environment too. With this diet, you get the best of both worlds!

When it comes to treating pain and chronic inflammation, my recommendations always have a strong emphasis on exercise (like we covered in chapter 5) and nutrition. A flexitarian style diet is a great recommendation for everyone as it's quite flexible and non-restrictive. Whilst each patient is treated on an individual basis, and no two cases are ever the same, it is something that is explored consistently.

We are not aiming for six-pack abs or bikini bodies. We are simply looking for a way to eat and exercise your way to health in order to avoid pain and reduce inflammation caused by excessive weight or poor diet. The overall aim is to allow patients to have a feasible and healthy way to clean living in order to keep them fit and healthy without removing meat from their diet entirely. Sometimes, people jump in and end up dropping out of an eating regime (or diet) because they feel restrictive and that's why it is always important to remember the philosophy stated at the start of this chapter – everything in moderation!

A Flexitarian diet is great because:

- We have an abundance of unprocessed plant-based foods that we can access easily. This includes fruit, vegetables, wholegrains, legumes, and nuts. They are all filled with nutrients and can help our body heal from injury and pain.

- You can minimize your intake of processed foods. This means that your meals are generally healthier and you are avoiding processed meats and added sugars and salt.
- You get to use olive oil, which is a great tasting, healthy oil. As a result, you should avoid refined oils such as sunflower oil, palm oil, canola oil, and corn oil.
- You can continue to have dairy products in moderation and can even focus on healthier dairy products such as Kefir and other probiotics.
- You have the flexibility to include red meats into your diet in moderation.

In addition to following a Flexitarian diet, it is also important to exercise frequently and limit your alcohol intake as this can also lead to inflammation.

**Understanding Metabolic Syndrome**

Metabolic syndrome is the name for a group of risks that increases your chances of heart disease, stroke, and diabetes. Metabolic means the processes that occur as part of your body's natural function but having metabolic syndrome indicates that your body is at an increasing risk of developing a long-term disease.

You are more likely to suffer from a health condition, like the ones listed above, if you have:

- Low Cholesterol Levels
- High Blood Pressure
- High Fasting Blood Sugar
- Obesity
- High Triglyceride Levels

If your body is not functioning correctly due to metabolic syndrome, you may also find that you suffer from increased and chronic pain.

Insulin produced in the body is essential for controlling the sugars in our blood. It tells the cells in our body to absorb the glucose in our blood. It also helps us to store fat when the body does not require more energy. Without this natural insulin, our body stops controlling energy absorption and blood sugar to the best of its ability, and this can make us sick. People with diabetes are often unable to produce insulin to control energy and glucose. They either need to control this by following a healthy diet or they need to take medicines prescribed by a doctor, which includes insulin. Keeping a healthy insulin level is extremely important in people who suffer from chronic pain as pain is often more severe in diabetes sufferers. Maintaining a healthy diet can improve that and it can also reduce the risk of you having diabetes if you don't already have it.

## Intermittent Fasting

Intermittent fasting is becoming increasingly popular as a way to lose weight but it can also assist when you're trying to control chronic illness. Intermittent fasting is when you consider the 24 hours in each day and you choose consecutive eating hours, but you don't eat outside of those hours. Let's say you eat 8 hours each day, between 8:00 and 16:00. You would not eat outside of those hours but you can eat within those hours. There are many variations of the diet but this is the general idea. Some people choose to control their diet further by controlling their calorie or fat intake during their eating hours. Intermittent fasting boosts your immune system too and can help you feel more energetic. It can also aid tissue health, improve your physical performance, and reduce your chances of diabetes. As it focuses on weight loss, it can also help to combat obesity.

## What's in Your Gut?

Our gut health is important as the gut function helps to balance out many parts of the body. The function of the gut is to balance the bacteria and the organs in your gut work together to help us eat and digest food. Within our gut, we have the esophagus, stomach, and intestines which all break down our food and process it so that it's distributed well. Things like bacteria and viruses are expelled while nutrients are distributed throughout the body to the places they are most needed.

Our gut is linked to stress, and as stress is linked to chronic pain, so is our gut. We can improve our gut health by many things, including diet and regular exercise. As you know, these things can also help us maintain a healthy back.

Many studies have recently found links between gut microbes and diseases which attack the body's immune system, such as rheumatoid arthritis, which is a chronic inflammatory disorder resulting in stiffness, swelling, and chronic pain within your joints.

Throughout this chapter, we've discovered just how important nutrition is when maintaining a healthy back. We've explored how we can improve our back issues, or even our back from injury or pain. There is a correlation between nutrition, health, and exercise, and each is equally important when combatting low back pain. It is certainly worthwhile trying out some of the dietary recommendations in this chapter, especially if you need to lose weight or eat healthier. The Flexitarian diet is a great place to start as it offers you flexibility when it comes to eating meat.

Next, we will review natural remedies and supplements that can help you nurse your back to health or prevent pain from occurring in the first place. Before you move on, have a think about some different ways in which you change your diet for the better and remember – everything in moderation. This philosophy includes exercise, so take it slow!

# 7

# NATURAL REMEDIES AND SAVVY SUPPLEMENTS FOR LOW BACK PAIN

If you suffer from low-back pain, there are so many remedies and preventative measures you can consider if you want to improve your condition. Of course, exercise, diet, and complementary therapies are not the only way to remedy or prevent low back pain. There are some natural remedies and supplements available that can improve your general back health along with many other health benefits. Considering natural remedies and supplements is a much better option than medication and it can be just as effective. They can also be a long-term solution whereas medication, especially pain relief and those with addictive properties, is not always the best long-term option.

Throughout this chapter, we will review different herbs and explore their functionality. We will also investigate the benefits of aromatherapy and supplements, so that you can form a well-rounded holistic care strategy to manage your low-back pain effectively in a way that suits you best. By the end of this chapter, you will have a broader understanding of the natural remedies and supplements that will help you improve your back pain, and you'll certainly be on the right path to a happier, pain free life.

## Herbs for a Healthy Back

We have access to a wide range of herbs that often have healing properties. Let's look at six of the herbs available that have specific properties that will aid back health:

**1. Willow Bark:** This is originally from central and southern Europe and has been used for thousands of years to treat pain and inflammation. It is said to work in a similar way to Ibuprofen. White willow bark, in particular, has analgesic properties. It also contains antioxidants and is known to boost the immune system. It can be used as an antiseptic to relieve arthritis and can even reduce fevers. White willow bark has been prescribed by experienced healthcare professionals to those who suffer from chronic low-back pain and headaches as sufferers have reported significant pain reduction.

**2. Boswellia Trees**: This is another anti-inflammatory ingredient and is known to treat all kinds of conditions that result in inflammation, like arthritis. It is native to India, the Middle East, and some parts of Northern Africa. Extracts from the tree are often used in natural remedies and supplements as it can regulate the immune system, reduce joint pain, and speed up the healing process. Boswellia trees are sometimes referred to as Frankincense, and in addition to helping with low-back pain, they help to fight against autoimmune diseases and cancer.

**3. Sour Cherries**: They are an antioxidant-rich fruit that can help with circulation and nerve function. Sour cherries also have anti-inflammatory properties, so if you consider this in addition to them helping with nerve function and circulation, you can certainly see how they help with low-back pain. They also help to fight against bad cholesterol and are believed to help improve asthma symptoms. They have also been linked to cancer prevention.

**4. Ginger**: There are many benefits to ginger. It is known for having therapeutic properties for arthritis sufferers and also works against pain and inflammation. Ginger is a relaxant and analgesic, so it improves blood circulation which helps to alleviate pain. Ginger can also improve sciatic pain and many people take ginger in their tea to make it more palatable. Ginger is a natural blood thinner, so you do need to take caution. Too much of it can also cause stomach issues.

5. **Nettles:** Nettles contain many nutrients and antioxidants and they have been used in herbal medicine for a long time. They can help cells and tissues heal within the body and have anti-ageing properties too. Reducing inflammation within joints and muscles in the body often results in pain relief too. Nettles can also reduce hay fever symptoms and lower blood pressure, which can improve our general health.

6. **Turmeric:** Turmeric also has anti-inflammatory effects and works well against low-back pain due to its natural pain relief properties. It has medicinal properties as it contains bioactive compounds which boosts your immune system and can improve arthritis symptoms. It can improve your metabolism, cancer, and various degenerative conditions. Turmeric can also improve your brain function and memory as well as lower the risk of heart disease. The recommended daily dosage for turmeric for those who suffer from low back pain is 1000-2000mg.

The commonality between all six herbs listed above is their anti-inflammatory properties and their ability to work as a pain reliever when it comes to low back pain. Depending on whether your pain is muscular, nerve-related, tendon, or disc related, could depend on what herbs you choose to try. It is recommended that you always speak to a professional when trying out herbal remedies, as they may be able to suggest the best way forward. Extracts from the herbs sometimes come in powder, solid, resin, or even liquid, so they can be used in many different ways depending on your symptoms. They can also give you advice on side effects and the recommended daily allowance for each herb.

**Top Dietary Supplements for Pain Relief**

Now, let's move onto dietary supplements that can support your pain relief. Most of these supplements will also be good for your general health and will help to boost your immune system. Such supplements can make you feel good, improve your well-being, and leave you feeling more energized. Let's start by looking at the benefits of Vitamin D.

**Vitamin D**

Of course, you have heard of Vitamin D already but *did you know there are different types of Vitamin D?* Vitamin D2 is one variation but we're going to be focusing on Vitamin D3. This is the natural form of Vitamin D, which we can even produce ourselves by absorbing sunlight. This suppresses inflammation within the body and is effective in alleviating pain intensity. Studies have found that vitamin D supplements have helped sufferers of chronic pain conditions, such as fibromyalgia. It is also linked with healthy bones and aids lung health which can assist with blood flow/circulation speeding up the healing process of soft tissues. Again, speaking to healthcare professionals can help you work out levels and dosage of supplementation. The recommended daily dosage for vitamin D if you're suffering from back pain is 1500 IU - 5000 IU.

**Omega 3 Fish Oil or Flaxseed Oil**

Omega 3 is often referred to as Fish Oil because this is ultimately where Omega 3 comes from. It is a form of fatty acid but it is healthy and is linked to reducing heart disease, ensuring healthy bones, and lowering inflammation within the body. Any product that reduces inflammation is going to relieve pain but be careful if you have high-blood pressure or take blood-thinning medication as this can have a negative impact. If you don't eat any animal products, you can use flaxseed oil and walnuts as these will provide you with some omega 3 benefits. It's not exactly the same as these alternatives do not provide this at the same level as fish oil. The recommended daily dose of Omega 3 fish oil for those with low back pain is 2000mg of combined EPA and DHA. If you choose the flaxseed oil alternative, the recommended daily dose for those with low back pain is also 2000mg.

## Turmeric and Curcumin

Turmeric has been mentioned already in the herbs section of this chapter so we're already aware of some of its benefits. Turmeric and curcumin are excellent at relieving arthritis pain symptoms due to the anti-inflammatory properties in each of these. Due to the levels of curcuminoids contained in supplements, in comparison to simply using turmeric spice, the supplement is much more effective and efficient. This means the results can be more noticeable at an earlier stage. The recommended daily dosage for turmeric and curcumin is 1000-2000mg.

In relation to supplements, you should always speak to a health or medical professional before taking steps to supplement part of your diet. This way, you can make an informed decision based on the facts and advice of a professional. If you do take medication or have health issues, this is extremely important because there can be side effects.

## CBD Oil

There has been a buzz surrounding CBD oil as of late, and many patients who suffer from insomnia and chronic pain symptoms try this before they seek medical advice or attention. Although it does have anti-inflammatory properties, and people with sleep and pain symptoms have reported positive results, more research needs to be done when it comes to CBD oil and its effects. The positives about CBD oil is that it has been reported to alleviate pain symptoms and it can reduce depression and anxiety too. It has also been linked to reducing cancer-related symptoms. It may have neuroprotective properties that could be used to help neurological disorders such as epilepsy, and there have also been signs to indicate it can improve acne. However, it is still early days.

There are many other health benefits that are being explored in relation to CBD oil but what we do know from recent studies is that there are many side effects including fatigue and diarrhea. It can also impact your weight and eating habits. It is really important to seek medical advice if you are considering using CBD oil as an alternative source. There is a chance it can cause liver toxicity, so usage should always be monitored. Even though it's considered safe at present, it can prevent other medications from working correctly.

**Over-the-skin Medical Patches**

Over-the-skin medical patches are readily available over the counter but many people make rookie mistakes when using these items for low back pain relief because they are not a hundred percent sure of how to use them, so let's discuss this further.

It is important to know that you should never mix icy creams or hot creams with over-the-skin medical patches. That's because many people have suffered adverse skin reactions as a result of doing this.

While some medical patches with a higher percentage of pain relief are convenient, they do require medical prescriptions. Lidocaine patches of 5% are typically available at the counter. They should never be worn for over 12 hours and it's still suggested that you speak to a medical professional about this as they can advise you on how to use them best. It is best not to rely on pain medication for long periods of time and this includes patches. Remember, the pain-relief is soaked into your bloodstream in order to relieve the pain. There are also common side effects to consider, such as burning or discomfort around the patch area, and redness or swelling to the skin underneath the patch.

Supplements should only be used if absolutely necessary. Before you consider any of the supplements discussed in this chapter, it is best to master the habits of exercise and eating/altering your diet for anti-inflammatory purposes. You owe it to yourself to do things in the healthiest and safest way possible before exploring alternatives. Ultimately, this means doing things in the most natural way – through a suitable diet and exercise. This isn't something you have to do alone as you can consider your options by exploring the topics discussed in this book. As mentioned earlier, you should seek healthcare or medical advice from health/medical professionals who will gladly provide you with the information you need.

Things are about to get exciting in the next chapter. It is all about you and mastering your own master plan for back health. *Are you ready to live your best life, with a pain free back?* Let's do this!

# 8

# FIRST-RATE MASTER PLAN FOR BACK HEALTH

You've made it to chapter 8 and this is where things really begin to come together. In this chapter, we are going to work on your week-to-week plan of action that ensures you maintain a healthy back. Your plan will consist of exercise recommendations and self-care activities that leave you feeling energized. Most importantly, you will consistently work towards improving and enhancing your back health, so you can live an active, happy, and healthy life. This includes living with a pain free back. We will also talk about signs and symptoms that you may need to look out for.

Just a couple of points to note before we begin:

- Stretching exercises are detailed in chapter 9 of this book.

- Strengthening exercise are detailed in chapter 10 of this book.

It is important that if you suffer from radicular symptoms, central stenosis, and disc herniations, you get advice from a medical professional before you start taking part in any physical activities, including the exercises from this book. This ensures you are able to avoid further aggravation and ensures your safety.

Let's dive straight in...

**Week 0 - Week 1 – *Time to Heal***

This first week focuses on active rest. Although you should avoid being completely bed-ridden, we should be looking at getting you up and walking at least once every hour. Sitting or lying down excessively can make your muscles stiff, which can result in your movement attempts becoming more difficult and more painful. Regardless of this, it's still important that you move.

Each day this week, you should:

- Rest to help your injury heal but ensure you walk around at least once in an hour.
- Utilize ice packs and ice the injured area for 10 minutes, followed by 20 minutes of rest each day. For optimal ice therapy, try wetting a towel

with cold water, wringing out the majority of water, and placing it directly on the affected region for cold compression.

- Start out with the first 5 stretching exercises from chapter 9, if possible, but only go to a tolerable movement range. Hold at that position but ensure you listen to your body. Don't push it! Remember, some movement is better than no movement.
- Perform 1-2 sets of these exercises every other day as you should take a day of rest in-between. Start by holding each for around 30 seconds. You can then follow on from this to build it up to around 45 seconds if you can

The idea of week 0-1 is to ensure you are healing but still moving too. Using the ice packs, resting, and completing some low-impact stretches can make a difference to your recovery.

**Week 2 - Week 3 – *Building but Staying Cautious***

It is still important that you don't overexert yourself at this early stage. You should continue working on the first 5 stretches and check in with your body regularly – *do you think your body is ready to commit to all the stretching exercises?*

By the time you are at week 2, you should:

- Already be able to perform 1-2 sets of stretching exercises, holding for 45 seconds each.
- Still be taking a day of rest in between.
- Still be using the ice packs on your injury, followed by the recommended rest period (detailed in week 0-1). You should do this daily or at least every other day (the day you exercise).

If you are doing this already and your back pain has improved by 50-60%, you may:

- Add the first 3 exercises from the strengthening program outlined in chapter 10 to your regime. You should perform 6-8 repetitions beginning with 1 set.
- Add a walking regimen to your recovery schedule. Start by walking for 10 minutes but gradually increase this to 30 minutes each day.

Depending on how well your recovery is, you should be adding a walking regime at this stage either way. Walking is so important when recovering from a low back injury because it helps to strengthen the back muscles in your spine which can prevent low back pain and help you maintain a strong, healthy back in the future. Building on your current regime is a great way to help you heal but also improve the motion range and strength of your muscles.

Walking is also a cardio activity that helps your muscles, tendons, and ligaments heal within the body. Cardio exercises not only help you maintain a healthy heart but they also increase blood flow which quickens up the healing process.

**Week 3 - Week 4 –** *Keeping the Momentum*

At weeks 3-4, you should be starting to notice the improvement in relation to pain. Although you're still in the early stages of recovery and need to be careful, you should also keep the momentum up. Of course, you still need to listen to your body but at this point you should be:

- Performing all stretching exercises outlined in the exercise chapter. You should be completing 1-2 sets with 45-second holds.
- Incorporating all strengthening exercises from the exercise chapter and performing 1-2 sets of 8-10 repetitions.
- Still icing your injury every other day followed by the recommended rest period.
- Following your walking regime.

- Still having a day of rest in between your exercise routine.

Keeping yourself motivated isn't always easy. If you struggle with motivation, here are four strategies to help you stay on track:

- Write down 5 reasons why you want a healthy back or why back health is important to you. Write them down in a persuasive way, so you can see the real benefits of why you want a healthy back. Whenever you feel demotivated, revisit your reasons. You may want to write them on post-it notes and stick them on your fridge or in a place you can see easily. It will remind you of why you're doing what you're doing!
- Set small goals and targets to meet but make sure they are achievable. You should never set yourself up to fail.
- Think of a small reward for yourself if you consistently follow your regime. It can be as small or as extravagant as you like – it really is up to you.
- Join a community/support group. I have created a community on Facebook called Treat Low Back Pain Naturally with Holistic

Strategies Mastermind, and this is a closed community for everyone to share and support each other during this journey.

*You can also find the group at: https://www.facebook.com/groups/treatlowbackpain

Even though it's difficult to keep up with an exercise regime over a series of months, the long-term benefits of recovery outweigh doing nothing. You will suffer for longer periods of time if you do not attempt to heal yourself, and therefore, it's up to you to take action and keep the momentum going.

**Week 5 - Week 7 –** *Going from Strength to Strength*

If you're managing to complete the regime from weeks 3-4, you are ready to begin building on that further. By building on your current exercise regime, you'll be going from strength to strength when it comes to your lower back muscles. Keep doing the things you have already been doing from weeks 3-4 but make the adjustments below:

- Perform all stretching exercises but complete two sets with a 60-second hold for each exercise.
- Perform all strengthening exercises but complete two sets of 10 repetitions. You should

be really focusing on the muscle contractions here.

- Increase your exercise frequency to two days in a row followed by a rest on the third day.

At this point, you will be starting to strengthen those muscles in your back. It is likely that you're starting to feel great as you improve but it's still important that you don't overdo it. A full recovery is usually 10 weeks plus and then maintenance should continue after that. You should be contemplating at least 15 minutes each day to maintain your back health but this will help prevent future issues.

**Week 8 - Week 10 – *On the Home Stretch to Recovery***

Throughout this chapter, I've stressed the importance of not overdoing it when it comes to exercise. You will be noticing a difference by now when it comes to your range when stretching, so continue to do what feels comfortable. If things are still going well, you should:

- Add onto your current regime by incorporating the advanced stretching and strengthening exercises.
- Maintain your two days exercise frequency with a rest day on the third day.

**Week 10 Onwards –** *Ready for a Long-term Healthy Back Routine*

At this stage, the functionality of your back should be between 75-95%. You should have zero to very little pain, and any pain you feel should be at a manageable level. If you are still experiencing some pain and feel your back is at 75% functionality level, you should continue with the weeks 8-10 routine for another two weeks.

Once your back is at or close to 95% capacity, you can switch to performing the daily habits routine (below) as this will help you continue with your recovery and transition to your normal activities that you completed pre-injury.

**Daily Habits Routine**

If you are now completing the above exercise routine for weeks 8 - 10, including the advanced exercises, and are now pain free, it is important to develop a daily habits routine from 3 times per week to everyday.

As your routine is simple and only requires 10-15 minutes of your time, it can easily become part of your daily schedule. Even if you're super-busy, you can still make time to fit in 10-15 minutes each day. It is important to continue with low-back exercises as it will prevent injuries in the future. Further injuries may take a longer recovery period and you will need to begin from week 0-1 again. If you are serious about maintaining a healthy back, the best thing to do is to keep on strengthening and stretching your muscles in the long-term. This is the easiest and healthiest way to a pain-free back.

Now, so many people don't want to be tied to a daily routine, so if you have to miss a day or two now and then due to being on vacation, don't stress. Although it is recommended that you keep up with this as often as possible, you should still be forgiving. Sometimes, life happens!

**Your Recommended Daily Routine:**

- Perform 1-2 sets of Bird Dog, Side Plank, Curl Up, Hip Flexor Stretch, and Glute Stretch.
- For Bird Dog, Side Plank, and Curl Up, perform 10 repetitions per side for each set.
- For Hip Flexor stretch, and Glute Stretch, perform 45 seconds each set for each leg.

Your recommended daily routine isn't too demanding and many people who perform a daily exercise routine often find that they begin to enjoy it as they feel accomplished. The practice of yoga consists of strengthening, stretching, and breathing exercises, and is popular because it provides people with enjoyable exercises that give you time to think and reflect. The strengthening and stretching exercises provided as part of your daily routine can also be enjoyable and give you time to reflect if you allow them to, but they solely focus on your lower back. Spending 10-15 minutes isn't a lot to ask for the sake of a healthy back and happy life.

As with any routine, it is important that you stick with the program. To stay on target with everything, you should print out a list and check them off each day, so you feel accomplished. Remember, that as with all exercise regimes, it is normal to feel sore and frustrated but you're doing this for the greater good. If you put in the hard work, there is light at the end of the tunnel.

If during any of the weeks, you notice that the pain changes to sharp shooting down the leg or you have an altered sensation, do not do any more of the exercises. Seek medical attention as soon as possible as you need a professional opinion before you carry on. Based on my experience, the majority of patients who completed the program have achieved a pain free lifestyle and are able to maintain it.

This master plan is laid out for you so you can start your journey towards a pain free back. Next, we will explore some stretching exercises for you to follow the program laid out for you in this chapter.

# 9

# STRETCHING EXERCISES FOR A HEALTHY BACK

This chapter focuses on exercise because in many cases, exercises are the key to recovery. There are many benefits of stretching, breathing tempo, and abdominal breathing as they aid your recovery.

When exercises are suggested to back pain sufferers, many clients tell me that they need clear instructions on which ones to complete and how to perform them. That's why this chapter covers how to perform stretching exercises along with some helpful pointers for each exercise. There are many exercises that offer low intensity to advanced stretches as well as stretch variations to enhance motion range. With that in mind, I'm going to discuss progression for each exercise in this chapter too.

Stretching is an important part of ensuring and maintaining back health. That's because stretching helps to make our back strong yet flexible, so it can help us complete day-to-day activities while preventing injury.

It's important to remember that no exercise comes without risk and there are risks involved with stretching too. If you do not stretch properly, it can result in muscle, soft tissue, and joint damage. The benefits of stretching include the risk of injury being lower, an increased range of motion and flexibility as well as relaxation opportunities. You must warm up well before you stretch, and remember, stretching is a gradual process. Take your time and increase the stretch gradually over time and be sure not to overdo it.

## Breathing for Stretching

Breathing is important for back health too because it increases blood flow within the body and helps us to relax. The speed or tempo of our breathing also aids our exercise. When we're stretching, we should breathe slowly. As your muscles stretch, you should exhale or increase the intensity and hold the stretch.

Many people don't breathe in the most effective way but *did you know that there are many ways to breathe?* In this chapter, we are going to talk about two different types that can be crucial if you want to maintain a healthy back.

**Chest Breathing:** To breathe in the most effective way when exercising, you should inhale through your nose. Inhaling through the nose is the best way to get clean air into your lungs. Allow the breath to expand your chest. You should feel the diaphragm and abdomen expand too but they should remain soft. Hold your breath for a moment and then exhale through either your mouth or nose.

When you breathe in, the diaphragm squeezes the blood out from the blood vessels so when you breathe out, the pressure lifts and the blood vessels can fill up with new blood. This contraction causes the blood to circulate well and this action helps push out the waste products accumulated in the muscles in the torso. This pumping action is rhythmic and is often referred to as the "respiratory pump". This is particularly important when stretching as the increased blood flow to the stretching muscles can increase their flexibility. It also removes the lactic acid from them at a faster pace.

**Abdominal Breathing:** We all know how to breathe as this is something we do naturally. To breathe from your abdomen, you have to re-learn your breathing techniques. This is beneficial as it ensures you trade all the oxygen you breathe in for the carbon dioxide you breathe out, so you get a full exchange. As this type of breathing slows down your heart rate, it can help to improve your blood pressure by stabilizing it. If you have breathing difficulties, this method is great for you as it prevents air from being trapped in the lungs and can help to strengthen your diaphragm.

If you want to learn abdominal breathing, you should:

- Lay down flat but with your legs bent at the knees.
- Relax as much as possible.
- Put your hand on your upper chest.
- Put your other hand just beneath the rib cage, on your stomach.
- Inhale slowly and deeply through the nose ensuring that the air fills up your stomach. The hand which lies on the chest area should stay still as you are focusing on bringing the air into your stomach.
- Keep your stomach muscles tight but allow them to fall inward as you exhale.
- The hand on your belly should rise as you inhale but fall as you exhale.

You should practice this breathing for 5 minutes and repeat this several times throughout the day if possible.

You should increase your breathing time up to 10 minutes as you improve your abdominal breathing.

**Stretching Exercise Program**

**1. Alternating Glute Med/Max Stretch Straight Leg and 45 Degrees** – When you first start with this stretch, you should start with one leg only. Do this over a couple of days and if you can do this without feeling any pain or discomfort, you can begin to lift both legs. You can also speak to a healthcare professional if you want to ensure it's safe based on your condition. To complete the stretch, you should:

- Lay on your back and bend your knees. Ensure your feet are flat on the floor.
- For one-knee raise, slowly and gently raise one bent knee. For two-knee raise, raise one leg up at a time as lifting both can be quite a strain on your abdominal muscles.
- Use your locked fingers to draw it closer to your chest. Ensure the stretch is comfortable and try to keep your legs, pelvis, and low back as relaxed as possible.
- Hold the stretch. You should be aiming to hold for between 20-60 seconds.
- Lower your legs back to the floor, one at a time.

- If you are doing the one-knee stretch, you should repeat on the other side. It is recommended that you complete the stretch 2 times for each leg but take it slow in the beginning. You should start by doing this once per day, then increase this to twice per day if necessary.

- For one-knee raise, instead of raising to the chest, you can bring the knee to the opposite shoulder and hold it there to target different glute muscle fibers.

- **Doctor's Reminder:** While performing this stretch, some people may feel pinching in the front of the hip, and this can indicate tight hip flexors. If this is the case, try to stretch out hip flexors before doing this stretch. If stretching the hip flexor doesn't help, it is possible that this can be caused by other hip issues, which can sometimes be because of different shapes of the femoral head and hip socket. In this instance, maneuver to the position that allows for a comfortable stretch of the glutes.

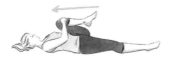

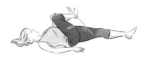

**2. Lying Down Pelvic Tilt** – This exercise can improve the alignment of your spine and posture. Many people with chronic low back pain have reduced control of their posture, so building the muscles can help to train this. To complete a basic pelvic tilt, you should:

- Lay down on your back.
- Push your pelvis backwards by pressing the small of your spine into the ground while exhaling.
- Inhale and push your pelvis forward. Relax your back and ensure you are only moving the lumbar part of your spine. Hold for up to 10-60

seconds. Start off at 10 seconds and build up the time slowly.

- When you've finished the stretch, relax, and then repeat the exercise.
- Once you have mastered this exercise, you can add movement to increase the intensity of the stretch.
- **Doctor's Reminder:** If you have underlying disc herniation, be extra careful with how you position the hip during this stretch. Some patients may find tilting the pelvis forward causes excruciating pain. If you experience pain aggravation do not perform this exercise. This exercise is beneficial for any patients with central stenosis as it helps off-load pressure for the spinal nerves in the lower back area.

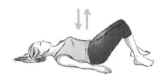

Try the advanced stretch (below).

**Pelvic Tilt with March** – To add the march to your pelvic tilt, perform the basic exercise (above) and when your pelvis is tilted, lift your foot off the ground and bring your knee towards your chest. Lower your foot back to the ground, then repeat with the other knee. The movement should be a controlled march, working at a consistent but manageable speed. You should ensure you keep your lower back to the ground and your pelvis forward during the march.

**3. Cat Camel (Cat-Cow Stretch)** – We have already talked about this stretch in chapter 5, but it is an important stretch that will assist your recovery. It is a very calming stretch that can help to improve your balance and posture. To complete this, you should:

- Get down on your hands and knees. Ensure your hands are in line with your shoulders and your knees in line with your hips.
- Keep your spine in a straight line and keep your neck long.
- Begin by facing down to the floor.
- Inhale and tilt your pelvis backwards. As you go into the stretch, raise your head so that you are looking straight ahead and point your tailbone upwards.
- Allow your stomach to drop down but keep your muscles right to support your spine.

- Hold the stretch at this point. You should be aiming to hold for between 10-60 seconds but remember to breathe. Ensure you breathe in before you begin the second stretch (the rounding of the spine).
- Exhale and lower your head so you are facing the floor again.
- At the same time, draw in your stomach and arch your back and shoulders so you are looking underneath your stomach. You should be aiming to draw in your tailbone.
- Take 5-10 slow breaths before you repeat.
- **Doctor's Reminder:** These two movements are my favorite movements to perform, but you should try to avoid any rapid and sudden movements throughout the exercise. Focus on your breathing during the stretch. For any patients dealing with acute episodes of disc herniation, you should focus more on the cat position as it helps off-load disc pressure.

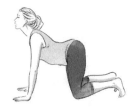

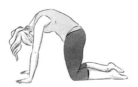

4. **Adductor Stretch** – This stretch is basically a tree pose but from a lying down position. As this is based on a yoga pose, it is actually a type of meditation stretch that can help improve posture, hip muscles, and tense shoulders. If you want a healthy back, this can help you stretch and strengthen your muscles. To complete this stretch, you should:

- Lay on your back on the floor or another flat surface.
- Straighten both legs and put them together so that the heels and toes are touching.
- Lay your arms and hands down by your sides.
- Bend one of your legs at the knee and place the bottom of your foot flat against the other leg against or just above the knee. Eventually, you should be able to place the heel at the top of the inside of your leg.
- Let your knee rest on the floor if you can – just follow the natural pull of gravity.

- Inhale and raise both arms above your head keeping the upper arms by your ears. Stretch upwards.
- Maintain the pose for 10-60 seconds or more but only if you are comfortable.
- Repeat the pose but swap legs.
- **Doctor's Reminder:** Be extra careful and cautious if you have a stiff adductor as progressing too soon in this stretch can do more harm than good. This is because the adductor muscle sits in a very delicate spot, and it can cause an uncomfortable feeling in the groin region when overstretched.

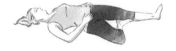

**Advanced Adductor Stretch** – Sit down on a flat surface and bend your knees out to the side. Bring the soles of your feet together. The side of your feet and ankles should be resting on the ground. Sit tall and hold on to the bottom of your shins. Remember to breathe deeply as you complete this stretch. Use your elbows to push your knees down towards the floor. Only do whatever is comfortable here, don't overstretch. Hold your stretch for 10-60 seconds and then release.

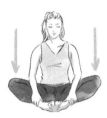

**5. Standing Quadricep Stretch** – This stretch is sometimes referred to as a hip flexor stretch and a wall mount quadricep stretch. It improves flexibility and can help you get your muscles ready for other activities such as yoga or running. The stronger the muscle, the less likely you are to suffer from imbalance. It can help with back health and also improve your range of motion. To complete this exercise, you should:

- Balance on one leg. If you are unable to do this unaided, hold onto the wall or a chair to help steady yourself.
- Bend your left knee bringing your heel towards your bottom.
- Use your right hand to reach for your ankle.
- Straighten your body, so that you are standing

up straight and draw in your abdominal muscles as you relax your shoulders.

- You will be able to feel stretch down the front of your thigh.
- Hold this stretch for between 10-60 seconds and breathe deeply throughout the stretch.
- Lower down your leg and repeat on the other side.
- **Doctor's Reminder:** This exercise is great as an introductory stretch as it is easily balanced. If you find yourself having difficulty when balancing, try drawing in your belly button. In addition, ensure you maintain an upright position throughout the stretch. Some people may have difficulty starting off this position and may experience muscle cramps in the hamstring as a result. In this case, stretch out the hamstring before pursuing this stretch.

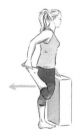

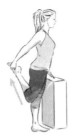

**6. Kneeling Hip Flexor Stretch** - This stretch is used to help you get your lower body moving. You have hip flexors at both sides of your body which allow you to bend at the hips. Hip flexor stretches can help people loosen up their tight hips and provide a deeper stretch as you lean into it. It is a great exercise to do prior to your strengthening exercises. It can certainly increase your flexibility too. To complete this exercise, you should:

- Kneel down on the floor on your yoga or exercise mat (if possible).
- Bring your left knee up and place your foot flat onto the floor, creating a 90-degree angle.
- Straighten your upper body, and place both hands on your left knee in front of you. This will help you to balance.
- Your right knee should be pressed into the mat while you extend your right leg behind you.

The top of the foot should be resting on the floor.

- Deepen the stretch by leaning slightly forward. You should look to hold this for around 20-30 seconds.
- End the stretch and bring your left knee back down to the floor and then repeat on the other side.
- **Doctors' Reminder:** Common mistakes that I observe from patients when doing this exercise are caused due to too much bending at the knee. This causes the knee to go in an unnatural position in front of the toes and can place excessive stress on the knee joints. Focus on keeping the front leg at 90 degrees and maintain an upright posture.

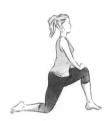

7. <u>**Wall Mount Quadricep/Hip Flexor Stretch**</u> – This stretch can also be completed against the wall, but in this position, a lot of pressure is applied on the hip.

Stand straight and push your shin backwards towards the wall. The closer you push your shin towards the wall, the more tension in the stretch. Don't overdo this – simply adjust the stretch accordingly. To complete the advanced stretch, you should:

- Bend your knee and place one of your shins against the wall with your knee on the ground.
- Lunge forward and put your other foot in front of you placing it flat on the floor, bending at the knee.
- Straighten your upper body whilst in this kneeling position.
- For a deeper stretch, raise your arms up in the air above your head and hold the stretch for 10-60 seconds.
- Repeat but remember to swap legs.
- **Doctor's Reminder:** This stretch can cause a cramping sensation in the hamstring if your hamstrings are feeling tight. If this happens, stretch out the hamstring before attempting this stretch. Another important tip is to ensure an upright posture as any forward or backward leaning of the trunk will reduce the effectiveness of the stretch.

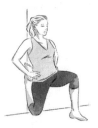

**8. Lying Down Single Leg Pelvis Rotation** – This exercise can help stretch your spine to help improve the muscles and make them stronger. Practicing this can improve your motion range. To complete this exercise, you should:

- Lie on your back and stretch out into a 'T' position. This means you should have your legs stretched out straight and your arms to the side.
- Throughout this stretch, you should keep your head flat on the floor. Your palms should be flat on the floor, so that they can support you.
- This stretch should be performed at a slow and controlled pace to maximize the benefits.
- Start to bring your left knee as you roll your hips to the right.
- Use your right arm to reach over so you can grasp the outer part of your knee.
- Gently pull upwards as much as is comfortable and hold the stretch for 10-60 seconds.

- Release the knee and roll back slowly into the starting position.
- Repeat on the other side.
- **Doctor's Reminder:** In this position, a clicking/gas popping sound from your lower back is normal. This simply means that the pressure is released from the spinal joints. However, some patients make mistakes, like over-twisting, which causes forced popping sounds. You should avoid this. If you are currently dealing with disc herniation, this position may not be optimal for you as it can place more stress on the disc itself.

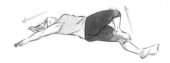

9. <u>**Seated Single Leg Pelvis Rotation**</u> - This follows the same concept as the lying down single leg pelvis rotation, except you form a deeper stretch by sitting upright. This strengthens spine muscles and increases motion range too. To complete this exercise, you should:

- Sit on the floor with your legs together straight out in front of you and keep your back straight.
- Bend your left knee and bring your left foot up to your right knee, and then cross it over, so the foot is on the floor next to your knee on the outside of the leg.
- Twist the torso to the left, so your body turns away from your knee.
- Place your left hand on the floor to support you and rest your right elbow against your left knee. Maintain a tall upright posture during the stretch.
- Hold the stretch for 10-30 seconds and then release the stretch, allowing the body to return to a neutral position.
- Repeat 3 times, and then repeat on the other side, twisting to the right.
- **Doctor's Reminder:** Ensure upright posture to avoid excessive rounding in the lower back.

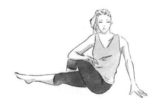

As recommended throughout this book, take it slow when it comes to stretching. Stretches should always be comfortable and should never cause you pain. Of course, you'll feel the stretch, which is usually a pulling sensation, but you should never push yourself too much. Breathe deeply when stretching and always start off by holding the stretch for a low amount of time and increase over time.

Now, it's time to move onto the next stage of this exercise program – strengthening exercises.

# 10

# BACK-TO-HEALTH STRENGTHENING EXERCISES

S trengthening exercises are a vital part of your ability to recover or prevent low back pain or injuries. Muscle strength helps you maintain stability in your lumbar area. It also ensures neuromuscular connection under tension and can optimize muscle engagement over time. Throughout this chapter, each exercise will focus consciously on activating muscle groups.

A typical human reaction to pain is to rest the painful area but when it comes to back pain, resting for longer than a couple of days can make the pain worse and slow down the healing process. When your muscles are strong, they can support your body in the best possible way and the risk of being injured reduces. When you follow a program of exercise, it is important that you stick with it as results take time.

Strengthening exercises can help to stabilize your spine and body. Your spine is under a lot of pressure as it supports your torso, neck, and head, as well as your arms. We put even more pressure on this when we bend or lift, so we should do our best to protect it. The mechanics of your spine help with the stabilization, and a healthy, strong spine can help you maintain good posture. If you suffer from acute or chronic pain in the spine or neck, spinal stabilization helps you remain pain free. Leaving injuries or problems with your spinal mechanics untreated can cause rapid wear and tear of the spine and the way it functions. The healing process in these cases can take a long time. It is important to seek medical advice, so you know and understand what the problems are and do everything you can to heal and protect your spine.

## Ankle Instability, Poor Posture and Poor Muscular Control

The ankle joint is commonly injured in sports due to ankle sprains which can cause chronic ankle instability. This can cause poorer neuromuscular control as well as poor posture, both of which are recognized as being a cause of instability in the spine and low back (lumbar) pain. The hips can also be affected due to the impact on their internal rotation. Evidence suggests that those with acute lateral ankle sprains are more likely to notice an alteration in their postural control than those without one. While most people believe they have recovered from their ankle sprain by resting their ligaments for two weeks, this isn't always the case. The reduction in swelling suggests that the ankle is healed but the ankle may not feel stable. This is because the ankle muscles that provide the stability are weakened, which means progressive strengthening exercises are required to help re-engage the muscles and return them to their previous health.

There are ways to test the stability of the ankle, and a common test is the Star Excursion Balance Test. It assesses your physical abilities and measures your balance by screening for deficits in your postural control as a result of musculoskeletal injuries. It can determine those who are at greater risk of injury by reviewing your flexibility, proprioception, and strength. This test is commonly used for athletes but can be used to check your neuromuscular control, postural control, and ankle stability to indicate if further strengthening is needed to build this and prevent further injury.

## Mind-Muscle Connection

The mind-muscle connection is when you are able to focus on the tension in a particular muscle that you are creating when carrying out exercises. It is a way to deliberately create contractions and helps you actively engage in the exercise itself which proves more effective. This is because your body is able to improve their muscles in a particular area.

The mind-muscle connection has many benefits. You can have better strength, a more balanced physique, and it can also increase your muscle growth as you use more muscle fibers and gain more muscle mass. If you suffer from low back pain or wish to prevent it, your mind-muscle connection can help you improve and heal at a faster pace.

Your mind-muscle connection can be improved if you focus your attention in the right place. For instance, if you are stretching your hamstring, you should focus your mind on this muscle and concentrate on how you distribute the weight of the stretch during your exercise period.

To improve your mind-muscle connection, you should:

- Turn off any distractions so that you can focus on your exercise.

- Visualize the muscles you are exercising.
- Make sure you warm up and concentrate on squeezing your muscles during the engagement time. I recommend squeezing the muscles when they are fully contracted for 3 seconds.
- Engage with the time you spend under tension during each repetition and slowly return the muscles back to starting position while engaging the muscles.

As mentioned in the earlier chapters, all exercise comes with risks so be sure to warm up first and also stretch to keep your muscles flexible. Completing a balanced workout has so many benefits. It can improve your mood and eliminate pain. It ensures your body is kept in the best condition and also helps you live a happy and healthy life.

Let's look at some strengthening exercises to ensure you have a healthy back for as long as possible.

**Strengthening Exercise Program**

Strengthening exercises are all about building your core stability as they ensure that every muscle and joint are coordinating and working together. Core muscles are those that make our body function in the correct way and spinal stability is key. There are 7 key strengthening exercises included in this exercise program and each of these contribute to improved lower back health. But before you begin, it is important that you understand that people can still have back issues, even if they have strong backs. The key is to exercise your back in the correct way – by ensuring we complete 'isometric' exercises. This is when the muscles are contracted and activated for at least 3 seconds but they do not change when it comes to the joints they cross.

**1. Bird Dog** – This can create further stability within your core muscles and surrounding joints. To complete this exercise, you should:

- Get on all fours, keeping your hands below your shoulders and your knees below your thigh. Keep your back neutral (this means you should keep a natural arch in your back and not force it into a straight position).
- Without moving any other part of your body, kick one of your legs to the back until it's straight.
- Ensure your back is in the neutral position at all times.
- Focus on engaging the glutes throughout your stretch.
- Hold the position for 3 seconds and then return to the starting position.
- Repeat with the other leg.

- **Doctor's Reminder:** This exercise is excellent for glutes activation as they are the foundation of building robust core strength. The most common mistakes patients make is lifting the leg too high, which causes the rounding of the lower back and twisting of the hip resulting in the uneven level of the pelvis.
- **Advanced Big Dog** – For an advanced exercise, you should straighten your leg and extend your opposite arm at the same time. Hold this for 3 seconds and repeat using your other leg and arm.

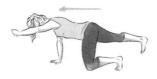

2. **Curl Up** – Many people perform the 'curl up' incorrectly and this can actually cause more pain and injury to your back. The curl up, if completed correctly, is great at strengthening your core muscles but you should be careful with this exercise, especially if you have back issues already. With this in mind, we are going to make some changes and do this in a way that

can help to stabilize your spine without causing issues. Take your time with this exercise, don't push yourself, and only complete it if you feel comfortable and feel no pain as a result. To do this, you should:

- Lay down on your back.
- Bend one knee, putting the sole of your foot flat on the floor but keeping your other leg straight.
- If you feel pain, straighten both legs and support your lower back by sliding your hands underneath in the natural arch before raising your knee again.
- Slowly, raise your chest and lift your head a few inches off the ground. Imagine you have a cushion under your head and roll your shoulders slightly off the ground as you push your chest up.
- Ensure you're in a fairly comfortable position that is not causing you back pain.
- Hold this pose for 3 seconds.
- Lower your head, returning to the resting position.
- Repeat this 5-8 times and perform two sets, resting in between.
- **Doctor's Reminder:** The goal for this exercise is to work on your core strength without compromising the lower back. Ensure your

head, shoulders, and body are aligned when lifting the shoulders off the floor. The most common mistake in this exercise is jutting the neck too far forward and causing strain. This causes incorrect activation of the core. Tucking in the belly when lifting the shoulder off the ground is also important to maintain core activation.

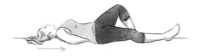

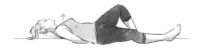

**3. Side Plank** – The side plank can help you strengthen your side muscles and the muscles in your spine. They are great for stabilizing the hip and pelvic area. To perform this exercise, you should:

- Lay down on your side with your knees bent.
- Push yourself up onto your elbow so that your body is at an angle. Let the arm rest on the floor.
- Put your other hand across your body and rest on your shoulder.
- Raise your hips so that you are only supporting your body weight with your arm and knees.
- Hold your position for 3 seconds before lowering the hip back to the floor.
- Do this exercise 3-6 times for one side, and then repeat on the other side.

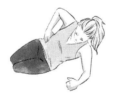

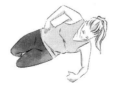

- **Advanced Side Plank:** If you are ready to progress with this exercise, rest on the elbow, but push up onto the feet rather than the knees. Keep the body long and create a full side plank. Your weight should be supported by your elbow and feet.

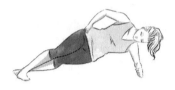

4. **Dead Bug** – This is sometimes referred to as abdominal breathing or tucking. This is known to be an effective exercise for people who suffer with low back pain. It works on building a solid core while keeping the lower back safe. To perform a dead bug, you should:

- Lay down on the floor, on your back.
- Ensure your head stays on the floor throughout this exercise.
- Push the small of your back into the floor by tilting your pelvis.
- Lift your right leg and left arm.

- Lay your left leg on the floor straight and raise your right arm overhead.
- Inhale deeply and feel your diaphragm inflate.
- Hold your breath and ready your stomach muscles by imagining that someone is going to put pressure on your stomach.
- Lift your right arm and left leg as if you are bringing them together while holding your breath.
- Return your left leg and right arm to the starting position slowly by counting 3 seconds, and then breathe out.
- Repeat but with the opposite arm and leg.
- Do this 3 times per side to start and work towards 6 times per side.
- **Doctor's Reminder:** The dead bug exercise is excellent for anyone who has low back pain. If you are unable to fully extend out the arm and leg into a straight line, simply extending by 20-45 degrees to start will help strengthen the core muscles. As you feel more comfortable, you can progress the exercise by using a block. This will allow you to have more engagement in the core.
- **Advanced Dead Bug:** If you are ready to progress with this exercise, add an object such as a small foam roller between your right arm and left leg and apply pressure to engage core

muscle. Follow the same principle as regular dead bug exercise starting by keeping the left arm and right leg extended. Take a deep breath from this position and keep holding your breath as you bring your left arm and right leg as if you are bringing them together, and slowly extend left arm and right leg back to starting position by counting 3 seconds and breathing out. Repeat the same process for the same side 3-6 times per leg.

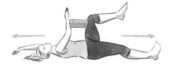

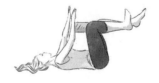

**5. Glute Bridge** – The glute bridge is an excellent exercise to help with tightness in your lower back and other back pain. This will both enhance your core stability and also activate your glutes. It is an easy, enjoyable exercise. To perform this, you should:

- Lie down on your back.
- Bend your knees to 90 degrees and place your feet flat on the floor.
- Start to elevate your hips upwards, and at the same time, squeeze your abs and your glutes.
- Push your hips up as high as you can without arching your spine. Aim to be in a straight line between your hip to shoulder and hip to knee.
- Hold the position for 2-3 seconds and squeeze your glutes as you perform this.
- Keep your abs and glutes tight as you lower your hips back down to the floor slowly.
- Rest, and then repeat the exercise 3-8 times.
- **Doctor's Reminder:** If you have been diagnosed with central stenosis, this exercise may cause discomfort in the lower back. If it's too uncomfortable, leave this one out and find another exercise to perform.

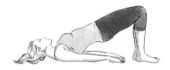

**6. Cobra Push Up/Upward Facing Dog** – For this exercise, we will begin by learning the Cobra Push Up, but for the advanced exercise, you can challenge yourself further by going into the Upward Facing Dog. This is a more challenging pose as you need to lift your legs and pelvis off the floor. This pose helps to stretch your muscles in your torso, including your shoulders, back and stomach, but it also increases your flexibility overall and decreases stiffness in your lower back. To begin the Cobra Push Up, you should:

- Lie down on the floor on your stomach, with your chest and thighs against the floor.
- Bend your arms and place your palms on the floor at the side of your shoulders. This is your starting/resting position.
- During this exercise, you should keep the lower half of your body, from the lower pelvis, down on the floor. Only your upper body should be lifted.

- Push up by straightening your arms or keep a slight bend at the elbow and raising your head and chest so that your torso is lifted.
- Hold the post for 3-5 seconds and then lower yourself back to the floor slowly.
- You should repeat this 3-5 times at first, starting with 3 and work your way up to 8 times.
- **Doctor's Reminder: The** Cobra Push Up and Upward Facing Dog are great for patients who suffer with disc herniations but you should be extra cautious as disc herniations may cause further issues. If you do these types of movements during the acute phase of disc herniation, do them lying down on the floor, on your stomach, looking up. You should take your time to progress any further in this exercise. For anyone with central stenosis, these two movements are not ideal as it will aggravate your back conditions. To perform these two exercises, constantly remind yourself to tuck in your stomach and engage your core.

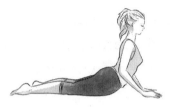

- **Advanced Upward Facing Dog** – To go into the Upward Facing Dog, you should lie down in the same starting/resting position. Push up into the cobra post by dropping your hips but raising the top half of your body. Breathe in as you lift the thighs and legs off the floor. Ensure the tops of your feet are pressed into the floor. Hold for 1-3 seconds while you continue to breathe. Lower your knees first and go back into the cobra pose. You can then repeat this exercise from this position.

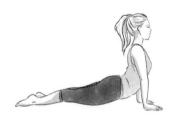

7. **<u>Side Lying Glute Med</u>** – If you want to keep your lower back healthy, you need to exercise your hips to prevent them from becoming stiff. Your hips, pelvis, and lower back are all connected and your hips are needed for daily movements. This exercise can increase hip and lower back strength, It is a simple exercise which can improve stability and strengthen your core. To complete the Side Lying Glute, you should:

- Lay on one side with your legs extended.
- Your hips and legs should be on top of one another, parallel with each other.
- Your feet should remain in a neutral position, so just relax your feet.
- Inhale deeply, and then on the exhale, raise your upper leg so it's just above your hip joint. You will feel the tension in your back and hips at this point so stop and hold the position for 2-3 seconds.
- Inhale as you lower your leg back into your starting position slowly.
- Remember, it's not a race. This exercise should be completed at a slow pace, and you should be careful not to raise the leg too high.
- You should repeat sets of 8-10 raises at first, but as always, take it slow and if you can only

manage 5, simply start at 5 and build this up slowly.

- Turn over and repeat a set on the other side.
- **Doctor's Reminder:** This exercise is great for isometric contraction in the gluteus medius muscle. If you suffer from acute low back pain, it is still easy to perform and will help you strengthen your lower back.
- **Advanced Side Lying Glute Med** – If you can do this exercise easily and feel you're ready for a more challenging way to strengthen your muscles, you can add a resistance band. Simply add a resistant band by placing it around both thighs and you'll feel the resistance as you make the leg raise. If it is still relatively easy, you can place the resistance band around the ankles instead.

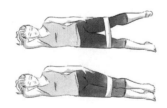

You've now reached the end of the strengthening exercise program and your journey towards a healthy back is now within your grasp. All that's left for you is to read my conclusion which sums everything up and brings this book and its ideas to a close. After that, simply head back to chapter 8 and complete the master plan for back health that we've outlined especially for you.

This will certainly lead you on your journey to reducing any pain and improving your low back health.

# SPEAK WITH DR. LEO CHOU

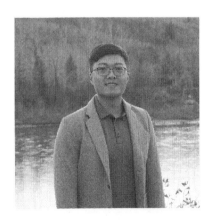

If you would like additional help and guidance on implementing these exercises to your daily routine or have physical limitations and underlying issues that prevent you from achieving optimal health, I welcome you to reach out to me personally and work 1 on 1 with me.

You can work personally with me, or you can go to my website for more information: www.drleochou.com

Once you are at the homepage, you can book your call. There will be a calendar with different times for you to choose from.

After booking your call, you will receive a confirmation email and there will be instructions within the email for you to prepare before our call. That way, we will have a more productive meeting.

Once on the call, I will discuss with you your current state, identify problems and situations, and see if I can help. If I am able to help, I will walk you through how it looks like to work together and come up with a plan.

The goal is to make you more informed and give you more clarity.

Visit www.drleochou.com to book your call today! See you there.

—

# CONCLUSION

Low back pain is something that people tend to ignore, especially if we don't really understand the pain and why it's happening. We seem to simply accept it as being general wear and tear but we don't have to, and we can make improvements or prevent injuries from happening. You can take charge of your low back pain, even if you're a beginner!

My aim, throughout this book, was to raise awareness and increase understanding of lower back and ensure that all readers understand the options available to them. We've explored the different parts of the back, the different types of pain, how diet, nutrition and natural remedies can improve the health of your lower back, and we've also looked at healthy back habits and treatments, including exercises for stretching and strengthening. This book has also provided you with a master plan for a healthy, pain free back so if you do suffer from back pain, you can overcome this without breaking the bank or spending hours visiting health-care professionals (although medical and healthcare advice is often advised, in order to receive a professional diagnosis). It is clear that you have everything you need to allow you to take the first step of your journey to a pain free back.

Sometimes, people don't take appropriate action to heal their back issues, and there are many reasons for that, including time and money. But even if you're super-busy or are unable to receive treatment imminently for cost reasons, you can maintain a strong and healthy back. Spending 15 minutes on yourself is a small price to pay to keep your back healthy because healing your back takes much more time, effort, patience, and money than simply taking early action. In the long term, 15 minutes is worthwhile, so make time and reap the life-long benefits.

It's obvious that many people allow back issues to escalate but preventing low back pain takes commitment. If back issues are not present or serious, you may feel the need to brush them off as unimportant but you are important and you should be committed to leading a healthy, happy, and non-restrictive life. Back health is something you owe yourself and the benefits are endless!

Commitment is a key component in ensuring good back health, and although exercise programs can seem daunting at first, they can really provide you with a new lease of life. You owe it to yourself to at least try the master plan in chapter 8 – you never know, you may even enjoy it. The question is: *are you committed?*

At this stage, I'm not going to go over the benefits of back health because we've discussed them throughout this book. The importance of back health is clear but only you can make the decision to follow through and stay committed to maintaining a pain free back.

Sometimes, if you want to make something part of your daily routine, you need to program your mind into believing it's a regular daily habit. This is so you perform your routine without thinking about it. To do this, you should:

- Schedule a regular workout routine and time – This will help your program become a routine.
- Set goals to help you stay motivated – Make your goals achievable and ensure they are set out in a way that will help you monitor your progress.
- Make your exercise a priority – You owe it to

yourself. Not everyone enjoys exercise, so ensure it becomes a priority and remind yourself 'why' you are doing this.

- Get involved with other active people – This could be something local to you, or it could be through social media or via an app.
- Reward yourself – This doesn't have to be anything extravagant but you could get some new fitness gear, celebrate achieving your goals, or upload some of your favorite tunes to listen to as you work out.

*Don't forget to redeem the free gift - **3 Daily Miracle Exercises: Have Total Control on Lower Back Health**. It can be redeemed at the beginning of this book and also at the end.

Staying healthy and pain free has many positive benefits too. It is a fact that pain brings us misery and for most people, all we want is a healthy body to enjoy life with our families. Maintaining a healthy, pain free back can help with both your mental and physical health, as well as increasing your energy levels. It can even bring you happiness because if we feel good, we are often determined to do the things that make us happy and socialize. This can help us externally too as we can become more focused on our family and careers without feeling restricted.

While low back pain is common, this book clearly shows that you don't have to be a low back pain sufferer and provides you with a path to help you overcome or avoid back issues. After many years of chiropractic experience, almost every patient with low back injuries or pain that I've treated, wishes they had acted sooner to prevent such problems. While it's human nature to put our own health last, especially if we're a parent, we need to reconsider the way we view self-care. For instance, if your back issues become so serious, you end up in bed for several days resting or need surgery, *who will care for your family?* That's why self-care is so important – a healthy, happy you, allows you to keep a healthy, happy family. I'm certain your family wants this for you, especially if you are their primary caregiver. You can't care for others if you are unable to care for yourself – that's a fact!

*Suddenly, 15 minutes or so per day, doesn't seem so bad, does it?*

In a world with increasing obesity issues, exercise is already recommended to ensure we are able to function effectively, stay fit and healthy, and lead an energized, healthy. and happy life, but we can only do this if we take care of ourselves.

Let's take a moment to reflect on a quote by Jim Rohn that I referenced in the introduction section of this book:

---

*"Take care of your body. It's the only place you have to live."*

— (BHATT, A. 2020)

---

We should all now see exactly what Rohn means when he says this. Often when it comes to our body, we don't always get a second chance. We need to care for what we have. We need to look after our body in order to maintain and sustain it, so that it can function in the most effective way possible as it is tasked with serving us throughout our lifetime.

This book has provided you with all the information and tools you need to maintain and sustain a pain free lower back. It is up to you to take what you know and make the change. You don't have to suffer from acute or chronic low back pain, and you CAN live pain free. *Are you ready to spend a small amount of time on maintaining your back health in return for a healthy and happy life?*

*What are you waiting for?*

Take responsibility, stay committed and start the program in chapter 8 now. Within 10 weeks, you will be wondering why you waited so long to begin!

Take Care!

*-Dr. Leo Chou*

**3 Daily Miracle Exercises: Have Total Control on Lower Back Health**

Jumpstart your low back pain recovery journey now!

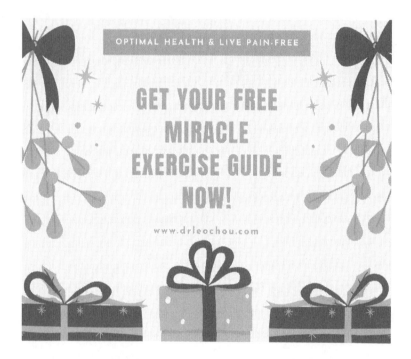

In this 3 Daily Miracle Exercises Guide, you'll learn:

- A shortcut exercise routine to help with low back pain in under 6 minutes.

- The most important key concept is to have a healthy low back.
- The top 3 habits you need to keep the pain away from the low back.

To receive your exercise scan the QR code below or visit - www.precisionperformancecalgary.com/gift

# ACKNOWLEDGMENTS

I would like to thank Janet Cooper who transformed my words into eloquent prose and made them easy to understand for readers through her engaging writing. And to Masha Pimas for drawing out such wonderful illustrations for different movements shown in this book. Thanks to my first mentor Evan Durnin, DC, Director of Peak Health Performance Clinic, for pointing me down the path of pursuing Doctor of Chiropractic Medicine. My thanks also goes out to my internship clinicians David Lee, DC, the leading clinician of South Riverdale Community Health Center, who has taught me the importance of team collaboration and communication. Additionally, Alex Lee, DC, lead clinician and sports chiropractic researcher from CMCC campus clinic, taught me effective patient interaction and clinical critical thinking. I also want to thank David Starmer, DC, for teaching me the art of chiropractic adjustments. I also would like to acknowledge Dr. Stuart McGill, Ph.D., for dedicating his life towards pioneering work on human body biomechanics and spine rehabilitation medicine.

My journey couldn't have happened without my parents' unconditional support, Tsui Feng Hung, and Jen Hsiung Chou. My gratitude goes out to my sister, Judy Chou, and brother, Monny Chou. And lastly, I must acknowledge my fiancée, Ann Tran, who has been endlessly supportive of my passion for my career, endeavor, and writing.

.

# REFERENCES

Bhatt, Ananya (2020) Quote by John Rohn, found in *25 Back Pain Quotes to Help You Cope.* The Random Vibez. (Accessed: 08/02/2021) https://www.therandomvibez.-com/back-pain-quotes/

Bhatt, Ananya (2020) 25 *Back Pain Quotes to Help You Cope.* The Random Vibez. (Accessed: 08/09/2021) https://www.therandomvibez.com/back-pain-quotes/

Frymoyer J.W er. Al. (1980) https://sci-hub.se/10.1097/00007632-198009000-00005 (Accessed: 08/10/2021)

Little. Jesse S. Khalsa Partap S. (2005) *Human Lumbar Spine Creep during Cyclic and Static Flexion: Creep Rate, Biomechanics, and Facet Joint Capsule Strain.*

https://www.ncbi.nlm.nih.gov/pmc/articles/PM-C1315282/pdf/nihms2927.pdf (Accessed 08/13/2021)

Marques Miranda (2021) *Diet, Body weight, and Pain Susceptibility - A Systematic Review of Preclinical Studies.* https://www.ncbi.nlm.nih.gov/pmc/articles/PM-C8237587/pdf/main.pdf (Accessed 08/11/2021)

Medicinenet (2021) *Low Back Pain (Lumbar Spine Pain).* Medicinenet. https://www.medicinenet.com/low_back_pain/article.htm (Accessed 08/09/2021)

Vora et al. (2010) Functional Anatomy and Pathophysiology of Axial Low Back Pain- Disc https://sci-hub.se/10.1016/j.pmr.2010.07.005 (Accessed 08/09/2021)

WebMD (2021) Back Pain in Pregnancy. WebMD. https://www.webmd.com/baby/guide/back-pain-in-pregnancy#1 (Accessed: 08/12/2021)

Block, D B. (2020) *Gate Control Theory and the Brain.* Verywellmind. https://www.verywellmind.com/what-is-gate-control-theory-2795208 (Accessed 08/14/2021)

McCaffrey, R., Frock, T. L., & Garguilo, H. (2003). *Understanding Chronic Pain and the Mind-Body Connection.* https://sci-hub.se/10.1097/00004650-200311000-00002 (Accessed 08/15/2021)

Weatherspoon, D. (2020) *What is Radiating Pain and What Can Cause It?* Healthline. https://www.healthline.-com/health/radiating-pain (Accessed 08/15/2021)

Duenas, Maria. Ojeda, Begona. Salazar, Alejandro. Mico, Juan Antonio. Failde, Inmaculada. (2016) *A Review of Chronic Pain Impact on Patients, Their Social Environment and the Health Care System.* Dover Press. https://www.ncbi.nlm.nih.gov/pmc/articles/PM-C4935027/pdf/jpr-9-457.pdf (Accessed 08/15/2021)

Jackson, Tracy P. Stabile, Victoria Sutton. McQueen, Kelly. (2014) *The Global Burden.* The American Society of Anesthesiologists. www.asahq.org (Accessed 08/16/2021)

Mayoclinic. (2021) *Biofeedback.* https://www.mayoclinic.org/tests-procedures/biofeedback/about/pac-20384664 (Accessed 08/16/2021)

National Institute on Drug Abuse (2021) https://www.-drugabuse.gov/drug-topics/opioids/opioid-overdose-crisis (accessed 08/24/2021)

National Institute of Neurological Disorders and Stroke (2020) *Low Back Pain Fact Sheet.* https://www.ninds.nih.gov/Disorders/Patient-Care-giver-Education/Fact-Sheets/Low-Back-Pain-Fact-Sheet (accessed 08/23/2021)

Spine-health. https://www.spine-health.com/ (accessed 08/24/2021)

Sweekriti, S. Traeger, A C. Reed, B. Hamilton, M. O'Connor, D A. Hoffmann, T C.

Bonner, C. Buchbinder, R. Maher, C G. (2020) *Clinician and Patient Beliefs about Diagnostic Imaging for Low Back Pain: A Systematic Qualitative Evidence Synthesis.* BMJ Open. https://bmjopen.bmj.com/content/bmjopen/10/8/e037820.full.pdf (accessed: 08/23/2021)

Ahorschig (2018) *The McGill Big 3 for Core Stability.* Squat University. *https://squatuniversity.-com/2018/06/21/the-mcgill-big-3-for-core-stability/* (accessed: 09/14/2021)

Arogya Yoga School (2017) *10 Health Benefits of Cobra Pose* https://arogyayogaschool.com/blog/10-health-benefits-of-cobra-pose-bhujangasana/# (accessed: 15/09/2021)https://www.homeremediesforall.com/food-remedies/ginger-for-back-pain.html#:~:text=Why%20Ginger%20Helps%20in%20Back%20Pain%20Relief%3F%201,tested%20for%20its%20therapeutic%20values%20More%20items...%20~:text=Why%20Ginger%20Helps%20in%20Back%20Pain%20Relief%3F%201,tested%20for%20its%20therapeutic%20values%20More%20items...%20

Evers, C. (2020) *How to Do Side-Lying Hip Abductions* https://www.verywellfit.com/side-lying-hip-abductions-techniques-benefits-variations-4783963 (accessed: 09/14/2021)

Mahaffey, K. *How to Do a Glute Bridge: Form, Workouts, and More.* NASM. https://blog.nasm.org/how-to-do-a-glute-bridge (accessed: 09/13/2021)

McGill, S M. (1999) *Stability: from biomechanical concept to chiropractic Practice https://www.ncbi.nlm.nih.gov/pmc/articles/PMC2485366/pdf/jcca00018-0013.pdf* (accessed: 09/13/2021)

POPSUGAR Fitness (2013) *What's the Difference Between Upward Facing Dog and Cobra Pose?* https://www.self.com/story/fitness-difference-between-upward-facing-dog-cobra-pose (accessed: 09/13/2021)

Rush Chiropractic. *Dead Bug: Core Exercise for Lower Back Pain and Core Stability.* https://nashville-chiropractor.com/how-to-perform-the-dead-bug/ (accessed: 09/14/2021)

Walker, N. *The Difference Between Upward-Facing Dog and Cobra Pose.* https://www.doyou.com/difference-between-upward-facing-dog-and-cobra-pose/ (accessed: 09/14/2021)

YouAreUNLTD (2018) *Understanding the Mind-Muscle Connection and Making it Work for You.*https://www.youareunltd.com/2018/10/05/understanding-the-mind-muscle-connection-and-making-it-work-for-you/ (accessed: 09/12/2021)

Advent Health Medical Group. *Sleep Hygiene and Back Pain.* https://www.thespinehealthinstitute.com/newsroom/health-blog-news/sleep-hygiene-and-back-pain (accessed: 09/04/2021)

Andrews, K. (2004) *A Healthy Weight for Healthy Back.* Spine-health. https://www.spine-health.com/wellness/nutrition-diet-weight-loss/a-healthy-weight-a-healthy-back (Accessed: 09/04/2021)

Catala, M. Schroll, A. Laube, G. Arampatzis, A. (2018) *Muscle Strength and Neuromuscular Control in Low-Back Pain: Eline Athletes Versus General Population.* Frontiers in Neuroscience. Germany. https://www.ncbi.nlm.nih.gov/pmc/articles/PMC6037821/pdf/fnins-12-00436.pdf (Accessed: 09/04/2021)

Cleveland Clinic. (2020). *Here's How to Set Up an Ergonomic Home Office to Avoid Aches and Pains.* https://health.clevelandclinic.org/heres-how-to-set-up-your-office-to-avoid-aches-pain/ (Accessed: 09/03/2021)

Healthline.com (2018) *Stretching: 9 Benefits, Plus Safety Tips and How to Start*

https://www.healthline.com/health/benefits-of-stretching#takeaway (accessed: 09/03/2021)

National Health Service UK (NHS). (2021) *Back Pain in Pregnancy.*

https://www.nhs.uk/pregnancy/related-conditions/common-symptoms/back-pain/ (Accessed: 09/04/2021)

Stenson, J. (2007) *Stretching May Offer Extended Benefits.* NBCnews.com https://www.nbcnews.com/id/wb-na21489011 (Accessed: 09/03/2021)

The Joint Chiropractic. *Avoid Back Pain While Cleaning the House.* https://www.thejoint.com/texas/hous-ton/katy-28013/avoid-back-pain-while-cleaning-the-house (Accessed: 09/04/2021)

The Mama's Physio. (2014) *Don't Let Breastfeeding Destroy Your Body.*

https://themamasphysio.com/dont-let-breastfeeding-destroy-your-body/ (Accessed: 09/04/2021)

Turetsky, L. (2020) *6 Exercises to Strengthen Lower Back and Core Muscles.* Backintelligence.com https://backintelligence.com/exercises-to-strengthen-lower-back/ (Accessed: 09/04/2021)

Dolson, L. (2021) *What is a Whole Foods Diet?* https://www.verywellfit.com/what-is-a-whole-foods-diet-2241974 (Accessed 09/05/2021)

Grajower, M M. Horne, B D. (2019) *Clinical Management of Intermittent Fasting in Patients with Diabetes Mellitus.* Nutrients. https://www.ncbi.nlm.nih.gov/pmc/articles/PMC6521152/pdf/nutrients-11-00873.pdf (Accessed: 09/05/2021)

Hillis Jr, R D. Pontefract, B A. Mishcon, H R. Black, C A. Sutton, S C. Theberge, C R. (2019) *Gut Microbiome: Profound Implications for Diet and Disease.* Nutrients. https://www.ncbi.nlm.nih.gov/pmc/articles/PMC6682904/pdf/nutrients-11-01613.pdf (Accessed: 09/05/2021)

Jabr, F. (2013) *How to Really Eat Like a Hunter-Gatherer: Why Paleo Diet is Half-Baked* https://www.scientificamerican.com/article/why-paleo-diet-half-baked-how-hunter-gatherer-really-eat/ (Accessed 09/05/2021)

Kress, R. (2017) *Stress, Inflammation, Immunity.* available at: https://www.rn.com/featured-stories/stress-inflammation-immunity/ (Accessed: 09/22/2021)

Lui, Y. Wang, Y. Jiang, C. (2017) *Inflammation: The Common Pathway of Stress-Related Disease.* Available at: https://www.ncbi.nlm.nih.gov/pmc/articles/ PMC5476783/ (Accessed: -9/22/2021)

Medawar, E. Huhn, S. Villringer, A. Witte, V. (2019) *The Effects of Plant-based Diets on the Body and the Brain: A Systematic Review.* https://www.nature.com/articles/s41398-019-0552-0 (Accessed: 09/05/2021)

National Heart, Lung, and Blood Institute. (2020) *Metabolic Syndrome.* https://www.nhlbi.nih.gov/healthtopics/metabolic-syndrome (Accessed: 09/05/2021)

Pahwa, R. Goyal A. Bansal, P. Jialal, I. (2021) *Chronic Inflammation. https://www.ncbi.nlm.nih.gov/books/NBK493173/* (Accessed: 09/05/2021)

Sissons, B. (2019) *Everything You Need to Know About Plant Based Diets.* Medical News Today. https://www.medicalnewstoday.com/articles/326176#benefits (Accessed: 09/04/2021)

U.S. Department of Health and Human Services and U.S. Department of Agriculture. *2015 – 2020 Dietary Guidelines for Americans.* 8th Edition. December 2015. https://health.gov/our-work/food-nutrition/previous-dietary-guidelines/2015. (Accessed: 09/05/2021)

Carter, A. (2020) *Using CBD Oil for Pain Management: Does it Work?* Healthline.com https://www.healthline.com/health/cbd-oil-for-pain (Accessed: 09/07/2021)

Chrubasik MD, S. Eisenberg MD, E. Balan MD, E. Weinberger MD, T. Luzzati MD, R. Conradt PhD, C. (2000) *Treatment of Low Back Pain Exacerbations with Willow Bark Extract: A Randomized Double-Blind Study.* https://www.amjmed.com/action/showPdf?pii=S0002-9343%2800%2900442-3 (Accessed: 09/08/2021)

Dumain, T. (2019) *Turmeric and Curcumin for Arthritis: Does It Actually Help Relieve Pain?* https://creakyjoints.org/alternative-medicine/turmeric-curcumin-for-arthritis/ (Accessed: 09/05/2021)

Gunnars, K. (2021) *10 Proven Health Benefits of Turmeric and Curcumin.* Healthline.com https://www.healthline.com/nutrition/top-10-evidence-based-health-benefits-of-turmeric#TOC_TITLE_HDR_11 (Accessed: 09/05/2021)

Healthy Women (2009) *Ease Chronic Pain with Fish Oils.* Healthy Women https://www.healthywomen.org/content/article/ease-chronic-pain-fish-oils (Accessed: 09/06/2021)

Helde-Franklin, M. Bjorkhem-Bergman, L. (2017) *Vitamin D in Pain Management.* International Journal of

Molecular Sciences. https://www.ncbi.nlm.nih.-gov/pmc/articles/PMC5666851/pdf/ijms-18-02170.pdf (Accessed: 09/06/2021)

Home Remedies. (2020) *How to Use Ginger to Relieve Back Pain.https://www.homeremediesforall.com/food-remedies/ginger-for-back-pain.html#:~:text=Why% 20Ginger%20Helps%20in%20Back%20Pain%20Relief%3F% 201,tested%20for%20its%20therapeutic%20values%20More% 20items...%20~:text=Why%20Ginger%20Helps%20in% 20Back%20Pain%20Relief%3F%201,tested%20for%20its% 20therapeutic%20values%20More%20items...%20* (Accessed: 09/07/2021)

Kubala, J. (2018) *7 Benefits and Uses of CBD Oil (Plus Side Effects).* Healthline.com https://www.healthline.-com/nutrition/cbd-oil-benefits (Accessed: 09/06/2021)

Levy, J. (2017) *Boswellia Seratta: Is it the Best Natural Cancer Fighter?* Dr. Axe. https://draxe.com/nutri-tion/boswellia/ (Accessed: 09/08/2021)

Medline Plus (2021) *Lidocaine Transdermal Patch.* US. National Library of Medicine. https://medlineplus.-gov/druginfo/meds/a603026.html (Accessed: 09/06/2021)

Raman, R. (2018) *6 Evidence-Based Benefits of Stinging Nettle.* Healthline.com https://www.healthline.com/nu-trition/stinging-nettle (Accessed: 09/06/2021)

Turcotte, M. *Health Benefits of Sour Cherry.* Livestrong.com https://www.livestrong.com/article/116111-health-benefits-sour-cherry/ (Accessed: 09/07/2021)

Appleton, B. *Breathing During Stretching.* Stason.Org. https://stason.org/TULARC/sports/stretching/4-7-Breathing-During-Stretching.html (accessed: 09/12/2021)

Asher, A. (2020) *Knees to Chest Stretch for Low Back Muscles.* Verywell health. https://www.verywellhealth.com/knees-to-chest-exercise-296870 (accessed: 09/13/2021)

Black, K. *Why is Breathing Important During Stretching?* Azcentral.com

https://healthyliving.azcentral.com/precautions-stretching-5880.html (accessed: 09/12/2021)

Clark, S. (2020) *How to Do Cat-Cow Stretch (Chakravakasana) in Yoga.* https://www.verywellfit.com/cat-cow-stretch-chakravakasana-3567178 (accessed: 09/11/2021)

Physiopedia. *Low Back Pain and Breathing Pattern Disorders.* https://www.physio-pedia.com/Low_Back_Pain_and_Breathing_Pattern_Disorders (accessed: 09/13/2021)

Physiopedia. *Pelvic Tilt.* https://www.physio-pedia.-com/Pelvic_Tilt?utm_source=physiopedia&utm_medium=search&utm_campaign=ongoing_internal (accessed: 09/12/2021)

Physitrack. *Spine Rotation – Single Leg Supine* https://us.physitrack.com/home-exercise-video/spine-rotation---single-leg-supine (accessed: 09/14/2021)

Quinn, E. (2019) *How to Do a Standing Quadriceps Stretch.* Verywell Fit. https://www.verywellfit.com/standing-quadriceps-stretch-3120301 (accessed: 09/11/2021)

THATfirst *Vrikshasana – The Tree Pose.* https://www.that-first.com/show/article/vrikshasana-the-tree-pose/ (accessed: 09/13/2021)

Thought Worthy. (2015) *Hip Flexor Stretch Against the Wall for Lower Back Pain.* https://www.thoughtworthy.info/BlogPost/Hip-Flexor-Stretch-Against-the-Wall-for-Lower-Back-Pain-187 (accessed: 09/14/2021)

YouTube. (2016) *Erector Spinae Muscles Stretches - Ask Doctor Jo.* https://www.youtube.com/watch?v=TovFXY7XYco (accessed: 09/23/2021)

Made in the USA
Las Vegas, NV
30 January 2022

42668968R00122